An Uplifting Experience

Cancer Is Not The End Of The World
It Just Seems Like it

Jan Guscott

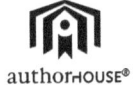

authorHOUSE®

AuthorHouse™ UK Ltd.
500 Avebury Boulevard
Central Milton Keynes, MK9 2BE
www.authorhouse.co.uk
Phone: 08001974150

First published by AuthorHouse 9/3/2009

ISBN: 978-1-4490-1217-5 (sc)

This book is printed on acid-free paper.

Dedicated to
Cancer Sufferers Everywhere

Acknowledgements and Special Thanks:

HOSPISCARE
Gina King
MACMILLAN NURSES
FORCE CANCER SUPPORT
R D & E HOSPITAL
Mr Ferguson, Dr Goodman
BREAST CARE NURSES
DISTRICT NURSES
CANCER RESEARCH UK
Irene Amos
Stephen White
Nicky Coombes
Publisher Gail (for her patience)
&
last, but not least: my husband **Simon** *(and son Nick)*
For always being there for me (in spite of everything!)
And all my friends, family and neighbours, whose support
and encouragement kept me going throughout this
challenging period.

(Hope I haven't forgotten anyone!)

{Some names have been changed in order to protect privacy}

[A percentage of sales will be donated to Cancer Research UK]

FOREWORD

The Spring of 2008 brought with it the greatest crisis of Jan's life. A breast lump was investigated and found to be malignant. Thus began Jan's battle to survive!

"An Uplifting Experience" is a courageous and life-affirming account of Jan's journey, written with freshness, honesty and lots of her natural humour. I believe that her book (whilst carrying you with her through her roller-coaster of laughter and tears), will prove to be an inspiration to all who read it.

As well as the total impact of the cancer on Jan, her family and friends, Jan records the highs and lows of everyday life, allowing her book to capture a period in "history".

Readers will begin to understand the incredible adaptability and scope of the human spirit – such is the total unaffectedness and honesty of her account.

I first met Jan in August 2008, four months after she was diagnosed with breast cancer. Her GP referred her to our community Hospiscare service, to provide support for Jan and her family during their life-changing experience with a potentially life-threatening illness.

As specialist nurses we work closely with other health care professionals and specialise in providing relief of symptoms, help with any concerns or questions relating to a patient's illness, treatment or medication, as well as providing practical, financial advice (and complementary therapies!!).

Breast cancer is the most common form of cancer in the UK. Age is an important risk factor and, statistically, 1 in 50 women under 50 years are at risk of developing it. (This incidence increases dramatically with age.) Thanks to writings such as Jan's, plus increased "breast awareness", screening and medical research, the condition is often now discussed earlier, and subsequent treatments are more advanced and successful.

Gina King
CNS Palliative Care

Contents

CHAPTER ONE

What a Boob!

No matter how hard you try, you can never be completely prepared....
for anything....

You go through life thinking...hoping...that all the bad things you read
or hear about will never happen to you. But of course, they have to
happen to someone, so this time they picked on me....

It all began nearly a year ago – I think. You don't start to mark time
if you don't attach much importance to the initial event. Something I
was soon to regret.....

Almost a year ago, I thought I could feel a small, almost miniscule,
barely worth mentioning lump, in my left breast. I asked my husband
if he could feel it, it was so small (the lump, not the breast!). After
finally getting his finger on the area in question he remarked that he
thought I had always had a lump there! That was good enough for me.
Even though I had often read that, on first discovering such things, one
should always seek out their GP, my husband's assurance was enough
to keep worrying thoughts at bay. He said that if I was worried about
it I should, however, see my doctor. Well that's what he says that he
advised. Maybe I've drawn a blank over that area because I don't want
to feel that perhaps, after all, it was my own fault that I am in this
current situation.

Anyway, time went on and I thought no more about it. I was always
aware of this little lump but, foolishly, not to the point that I was overly
concerned. Occasionally I asked him to see if he could feel if it was
getting any bigger, because I thought, perhaps, it was. "Hmm...maybe

a little," he confirmed. I started to worry just a little. But, stupidly, still not enough to do anything about it – like my husband could replace a doctor in these instances! I learned the hard way....

I seemed to be more impressed by the fact that my left boob seemed to be getting larger than my right boob! I had no idea why – I simply wished my right boob would do the same and "catch up" so I would look more "even"! However, a nice big left boob didn't concern me at all! Oh dear!

A couple of months later, I started to feel little twinges in my left breast near the nipple area. I wondered what was causing this. It always seemed to happen at the most inconvenient time, for instance, whilst at work at the law firm, sitting at the computer, trying to type whilst resisting the urge to scratch myself, hoping my twisted facial expression would vanish before anyone passed by.

After a couple of weeks I had to visit my local GP on another matter and, whilst I was there, I mentioned this slight pain. She was a fairly young, slim, fair-haired, pleasant lady who was quietly spoken. She asked how often I felt the pain and how long it lasted. I said sometimes it was daily, or every other day, and only for a few minutes at a time. She said nothing and pursued my other ailment. She was obviously not worried and I guessed she couldn't spend any more time on that matter because they can only deal with one complaint at a time in the alloted appointment time of ten minutes! I suppose I must have seemed more concerned about my other problem – a polyp which had to be removed and sent off for analysis. Again, that was good enough for me! If the GP wasn't unduly concerned surely there was definitely nothing to worry about then?

A week later I had the minor op. and a week after that I became yet more aware and concerned about the pain in my left breast. I decided to see my GP again. This time she examined it but thought it was quite possibly some kind of fibrous tissue, which would be nothing to worry about. However, she asked my age, and concluded therefore, to be on the "safe side", that I should go and have a mammogram at the main hospital some twenty miles away. She put me on the "fast track" which she tried to assure me was what she always did in these cases, just to decrease the time in which I could be seen, so there was no undue cause for alarm. This, kind of, satisfied me. She said to let her know if I hadn't received a hospital appointment within three weeks.

On the short drive home I found myself thinking, inexplicably, of Toby, our Springer Spaniel. He had had a bit of trouble with his paw a few months previously. The middle-aged, grey-haired vet diagnosed arthritis and thought there might also be an infection so he gave him some antibiotics to take for a week. A few months later the paw seemed worse, so I took him to the vets again. After studying Toby's paw the vet look concerned. He referred to the fact that we should have brought Toby in again much sooner if we had noticed there had been no improvement. Whoops! We're just no good in medical situations – for humans or pets!

He was delicately holding Toby's paw, examining it, whilst I was bent over the dog, who was fairly cool to begin with, but there was no telling how long that would last, so I tried to sooth him by stroking the shiney black and white fur on his head. Although he couldn't be 100% certain, the vet seemed pretty convinced our dog had a cancer lump on the underside of his enlarged paw. Well, it was pretty visible by now even to the untrained eye. I stopped stroking his head for a moment and stared in disbelief at the vet. My hand was motionless.

"Cancer?" I asked incredulously.

He said, due to Toby's age (13 ½), there was little point in amputation as long as he seemed to be enjoying his quality of life currently. I said he was – that's why I was so surprised at this relevation. He would still run around a field like a puppy off the leash taking his first taste of freedom (I had long since learned why these dogs are called "Springers" – just let go of the lead and I defy anyone to try and catch up with them as they "spring" off") And as for his appetite – he was worse than me for eating non-stop (I do like my food)! People must have thought we starved the poor thing the way he was always hanging around for more food!

I agreed to purchase a special "designer" boot for him to wear when he went out (apparently that was how they were designed now – bright silver with laces – cute). Little did I know how his life had been actually paralleling mine (except the designer boot!).

So there it was – I had to accept that our beloved pet (ours since he was seven weeks old, bought from an army Major and his wife in Surrey) had cancer. I just didn't associate pets with getting that kind of illness. Oh well. At least he seemed OK in himself and still enjoyed food and walks (or rather, runs!)

I was abruptly brought back to my own situation when I got "cut up" at the mini-roundabout near my home and blasted the driver of the white transit van with my car horn. The driver looked somewhat harrassed as he tried to manoeuvre his van around the roundabout to avoid me hitting him. Despite my feelings I managed to get as close as I could without actually hitting his vehicle. Now I can count on one hand how many times I've blasted my horn in all my 30+ years of driving! I'm usually a much more patient driver, as I am with most things. But for some reason I just had to let out a kind of.....frustration....and unexpected disappointment with the news I had just received. OK so nothing had been confirmed – yet. But still....

A few days later I had written confirmation of an appointment for a mammogram the following week. I was impressed, yet a little anxious. Either there was a very short waiting list or else they were quite concerned! Unfortunately, this co-incided with my second week at my new job at the Police Headquarters. Fortunately, they were very understanding and were with me all the way regarding time off for this nailbiting appointment. It also probably helped that my new boss was an ex-nurse and was able to advise on a lot of what to expect.

CHAPTER TWO

Expect the Unexpected

Alix, one of the other secretaries, a young woman in her mid-twenties, became aware of what the forthcoming appointment was for. When she found out, she commented on how, despite my "cool, outgoing, happy exterior", I must have been in turmoil inside. Though that might have been the case for most people, strangely, it wasn't for me. Well, not yet anyway. I obviously knew what I was going for and what the x-rays were on the lookout for but, for some reason, the gravity of the situation still hadn't really struck home. I wish it had. But I didn't have to wait too long.

Brilliant sunshine heralded the start of the following Tuesday afternoon. I was having breakfast whilst watching television and just happened to catch a news article referring to TV celebrity Trisha Goddard who had, just that day (or the previous day) been diagnosed with breast cancer. I didn't really want to hear that, anticipating that it would be mirroring my own situation.

My boss tried to make me feel better about my predicament by informing me that medicine was very radical years ago but now it is a "science" and they are not guessing – they used to be like butchers! Kind of comforting I suppose....

I decided to do as much research as possible about what exactly was involved in the process. I checked out medical websites in an effort to learn more about the procedures in order to "prepare" myself for what was to come. I was quite surprised at what I found out, without taking into consideration the fact that one shouldn't always believe what one reads: a mastectomy constituted 2 hours operating time,

5

7 – 10 days in hospital (slight exaggeration I later discovered!), hand-arm swelling possibly requiring wearing a plastic sleeve on the arm, no lifting for three weeks, no driving, tubes sticking out of your body (mind-boggling!), tablets for a year (or even five years), shoulder numb for a year/needing physiotherapy, support needed after diagnosis and after operation, possibility of reconstructive surgery at later date, and something about a cumfie! Not much then! I even discovered how the scars would appear on a breast after a lumpectomy; either horizontal or diagonal apparently.

Later that day I went to hospital, on my own, straight from work, leaving a couple of hours early. I spent half an hour searching for a car parking space somewhere amongst the large hospital's many car parks. I ended up parking in the main street half a mile away and was a little unsure as to which building I was meant to go in. Fortunately, I had had to take my teenage son to the same building a while ago so I was fairly certain as to which one it was. Once inside the foyer, I checked with the receptionist I was in the right building and she confirmed I was and told me where to go – in the nicest possible way!

I eventually made my way, quite confidently, up the stairs – well, why take the lift for one flight of stairs, I thought?

At the top, I halted and scanned the dangling ceiling signs and wall signs dotted all around. I obviously looked lost because a passing nurse asked if I needed assistance. She kindly pointed me in the right direction a few yards down the corridor. I eventually found the Surgical Outpatients' Clinic and reported in. There must have been about eight rows of six chairs each in the immediate area. Unfortunately, virtually all bar a couple of seats were taken. "How long am I going to wait here?" I wondered. I was bang on time, as I nearly always am for doctors, dentists and hospital appointments though, strangely, not always necessarily for job interviews! Don't ask me why. I relaxed on one of the two remaining seats, which was quite comfortable actually.

It was quite warm in there. There were a variety of people waiting to be seen. I noticed some women had their husbands or partners with them. There was even quite a young girl with her mother – couldn't have been more than 15 I'd say.

No-one spoke a word. You could hear a pin drop. It was like sitting on a train. People were either reading magazines or staring into space, trying not to look at the person directly opposite them – I was one of those. I didn't really fancy reading as I'd been on the computer all day. I wanted to give my eyes a rest.

They didn't rest for long. I was soon given a form to complete while I waited, which asked questions about my health generally, exactly where my problem was, did any of my family suffer from breast cancer, etc. etc. I started to complete this when a nurse called everyone's attention to apologise for the delay which was, unfortunately, about 45 minutes for a particular doctor. I felt so relieved she wasn't referring to mine! I finished the form and returned it at the same time as another female patient handed hers in.

Every time a nurse or member of hospital staff appeared, everyone looked up, hoping their name was going to be called. Of course, invariably the worker was just en route to some other part of the building. I counted how many people must have been due to be seen before me but of course, I couldn't really tell because there was more than one consultant on duty.

Anyway, after about quarter of an hour I was called – I was one of the lucky ones...in that respect at least!

I was shown into a small room by a nurse who told me to strip to my waist and put on one of the little gowns laid neatly in a nearby pile. I could put my own clothes and handbag in the little blue basket (which looked like it came from a supermarket) on the nearby chair. She told me to sit on the edge of the bed and the doctor wouldn't be long.

I tried to do as instructed as quickly as possible – who wants to be interrupted whilst getting undressed? So unsophisticated! Of course, so was the gown. Naturally, it was not immediately obvious to a semi-nervous, "trying to be calm" patient, as to which way round it was meant to go. And where were the holes for my arms? How did it do up? Oh yes – funny little velcro type patches. It went down as low as my waist, so I kept trying to raise the waistband of my skirt to meet the hem of it! I wanted to be relaxed and sitting on the bed when they came in - amazingly, I was. Moments later, the Registrar entered - a young, Middle Eastern-type gentleman with a beard, who told me his name, which I promptly forgot, though I remember it sounded quite interesting! He informed me that he would be dealing with me today as the Consultant Surgeon was not in. I tried not to look too disappointed.

I was instructed to lie down on the bed. They never seem long enough for anyone over 5'7"! My feet almost dangled over the end. He put on some gloves (clinical of course) and I had to remove my little gown and proceeded to have my breasts manipulated in every direction possible. I had no idea I was so pliable! As is usual, the female nurse had to remain in the same room.

After fondling, em, examining me, he told me he was just going to take some cell samples from my breast and promptly vanished into the next room to get a syringe etc. I was not a happy bunny. Still, he returned shortly (nurse still in the room) and warned me about the little prick I was going to experience! I had my own warning to give – I told the nurse to expect I was now going to talk a lot of jibberish simply to take my mind off what he was about to do. I looked away and did just that! She must have been used to it though and in fact encouraged me! In between the "rubbish" all you could hear was a calm "Ow...yes that hurts just a bit and...yes, that hurts too....so anyway, what I was saying was..."

After about an hour – OK, a few seconds I suppose – he removed the needle and apologised for the pain. He went away and the nurse told me to just lie still for a moment until he came back.

We continued the conversation I had begun whilst I was being stabbed! Only I like to think I was a little more coherent by now. She seemed particularly impressed by my line of work (I don't know why – I was more impressed by hers!)

"I would love to do something like that," she said, whilst organising the pile of gowns on the nearby table, "but I don't have your skills....you say you do shorthand?"

"Yes," I replied, "I think I'm the last person in the world by the way no-one wants me to use it!" I couldn't help my sarcasm. "But surely, don't you find your job rewarding?"

"Not any more...I've been doing it for six years now...I'd like a change..."

"Oh." I didn't know what else to say. I just don't know where we would all be without nurses. Maybe I should have said that.

The Registrar whose name I couldn't remember came back and told me that, while he was going to examine the results of this, I should go for my mammogram but that I also needed to attend for Ultrasound. This was all on a different level so he gave me a note to take with me, telling me to keep my gown on and take my little blue basket of clothes and handbag with me. This was all slightly more than I had expected but little did I know that worse was yet to come!

So off I trundled, self-consciously still wearing my little gown, along the many corridors, down the stairs, along more corridors, reading more signs up above and on the walls, searching for Letter F and the X-Ray department. I eventually found it. I walked into the small Breast Care Unit and handed my note to the fairly austere receptionist, holding onto my gown to make sure it didn't come undone.

"Been here before?" she asked, as if I were a criminal being interviewed by a judge at court.

"No," I assured her. I mean, what a question! But, of course, anyone with an ounce of sense would naturally have been there on a regular basis, but no, not me!

"Take a seat," she continued, not looking up, "someone will be with you shortly." I was willing to give her the benefit of the doubt and did as instructed. I recognised the only other people in the confined waiting area – a man and his wife who had been waiting earlier in the large Surgical Outpatients Waiting area. His wife looked even more austere than the receptionist. She was slim, middle-aged, with close cropped, silver blonde hair. Like me, she was adorned with a little gown. She had many lines on her face – perhaps she had had a hard life. Maybe she already knew the outcome of her situation. But whatever the reason, her facial expression certainly didn't invite conversation, unlike her husband – a large, middle-aged, cheery-looking chap.

I helped myself to a drink of water from the nearby machine and sat down again, trying to ignore the tempting skew-whiff bundle of magazines on the table next to me. I wanted to concentrate on the job in hand – or so I kept telling myself. The man's wife then disappeared. Moments later, her name was called.

"Oh, I'm afraid she's just gone to the lavatory," her husband smiled at the nurse.

"That's <u>my</u> luck!" I commented. He smiled back.

The nurse said that was no problem and she would come back. I had secretly hoped she would ask me to go instead, but, alas no such luck! See? That's just my luck too!

A little while later, I was joining his wife on a couple of seats in the corridor, awaiting my mammogram.

It was a narrow corridor in which our row of seats was set. Consequently, I found myself constantly having to bring my feet in to avoid the passing people traffic, then outstretching them for comfort before the next person passed by, which was never too long a wait.

Between the feet shuffling I opened my bag and took out a sweet that used to be called an Opal Fruit but for some reason is now called "Starburst". I kept adjusting my gown. Good – no-one could see my breasts before they had to! After a while I was led into a room to have my mammogram done (or "Dadogram" as my husband, Simon, liked to call it! Don't ask why!).

A friendly nurse instructed me to place my basket on a nearby chair and remove my gown. She then explained the procedure about to take place. I was prepared for a basic X-ray – I'd had a few in my time: sprained ankle, hairline fractured elbow, teeth - that sort of thing. I was, however, a little unprepared for this type of X-ray. She told me to lean into a large machine and place my right breast (the one that was apparently OK) onto a similar sized glass plate, holding onto a bar above. "Oh, I've seen pictures of these," I remarked.

"Yes, you probably have," she replied before advising me that my breast was now about to be sandwiched between two plates! I had no idea how flat a 38DD breast could go – until now!

"It may just feel a little uncomfortable," she advised before disappearing behind a window.

Moments later she called to me to hold my breath, which I did. Then I was told to exhale before she came out and adjusted the plates so that the edge of one was pressed hard against the middle of my chest wall. I give her her due – she did warn me that this time it might be a little more painful – and she was right.

"Wow" I queried, "If this hurts and this is my good one, what's it going to be like for the other one?"

"Yes, I'm sorry," she seemed genuinely apologetic, "I'll try to be as quick as I can with your other one!" and promptly disappeared behind the window again.

After this session was complete I was told to wait again in the little corridor outside, still in my little gown, to await my Ultrasound session. I did as instructed. After a few minutes, the seats immediately next to me became occupied by a blonde teenager and her mother, who barely said a word.

Eventually I was called into the little room opposite, so in I trundled with my faithful basket of belongings, ushered in by another nurse. There I was met by a very young male doctor seated at a desk staring at x-rays of round objects (well, he seemed young to me – I'm not as young as I was!). He finally rose from his desk and introduced himself but, again, I didn't really take in his name – I was more concerned with trying to see the x-rays:

"Are those mine?" I asked.

"Yes," he replied in a matter-of-fact fashion. The nurse told me to remove my little gown and lie down on the nearby trolley bed next to a machine that looked like a computer.

The doctor then came over to the machine and proceeded to cover a small, hand-held implement with a jelly-like substance, then told me to raise my left arm beside my head and turn my head to the right. He then commenced to use the implement to rub the substance around my left breast whilst the nurse stood the other side of the bed.

"Oh, this is like when I was pregnant!" I remarked.

"Yes, that's right," he confirmed, "they usually do this then..." he continued to manoeuvre the substance all around my breast (all the while staring at the monitor), this time with more pressure, and then surprised me by moving the implement to my armpit.

"Well, they didn't put it there when I was pregnant!" I remarked.

I could actually just about see the monitor myself if I raised my head a little but this didn't please him – he had to keep telling me to lay my head down!

Soon he stopped and explained he could feel not just one but two lumps inside my left breast and also one under my armpit. This was apparently my lymph gland area. These had shown up following these procedures so now he informed me that I would have to have more samples taken from these areas once I was injected with something to make the whole areas numb.

"When will you do that?" I asked.

"Now," he replied.

"Oh. I didn't think I was going to be "stabbed" any more today!"

Although not mentioned by name, these were obviously going to be biopsies.

I warned this nurse, as I did the first one, that she should expect me to talk jibberish while he injected me.

"Don't worry," she reassured me, "You'll be amazed at some of the things we hear in here!"

The nurse later told me I was, apparently, quite brave (and lucky!) to have all these various procedures carried out on me in one afternoon!

The doctor proceeded to show me long, tube-like implements about the size of tampons (but stronger, of course!) that he would use for this, including the sections near the bottom that were used to "capture" the sample, making a slight sudden noise as the action took place. He informed me that he would give me advance "warning" just before that happened and that there would be minimal discomfort.

He proceeded to inject me with a "numbing" substance which I remember felt slightly cold. It wasn't long before I felt nothing in those areas. So then he proceeded to cut into my breast and insert those tube things into it.

"It will go quite a way in," he advised.

"OK" I said.

I didn't really feel too much (fortunately!). I just stared at the bare ceiling and let him get on with it.

"This is like being at the dentist!" I commented, "Maybe you should put something on the ceiling for us to look at!"

I got the impression not many patients talked whilst this was going on.

Then I got his advised warning:

"OK, it's going to make a click now," he said.

A split second later I heard and felt a "bang" from inside my breast! Some warning – a split second – not much time to prepare! The feeling wasn't too bad though – probably due to the numbness. All the same, I was aware something was going on inside my body but, well, if it ended up letting me know the full extent of what was happening there, it must have been a good thing to go through.....mustn't it?

The next thing I knew, he was telling me he was going to do this three more times from different areas, as this would be better than me having to come in again for more biopsies.

"OK", I said. What else could I say? He was the doctor....

A few minutes later it was over. The nurse plastered my left boob and underarm with various bandages and plasters.

I was then taken to a little cubicle by the "mammogram" nurse just next to the dreaded mammogram machine, where I was told to get dressed. I'd only got as far as putting my bra back on when someone tried to come in (a nurse presumably? Hopefully!) Fortunately the door was locked and they apologised and went away. I don't know who was more embarrassed!

I soon got dressed, left the basket with little gown on the seat there, picked up my handbag and went through the door on the opposite side as instructed. This opened out onto a little corridor (the smallest one yet!) which led back to the Breast Care Unit reception. The nurse eventually appeared and gave me some paperwork to take with me back to the first level reception. We bid a cheery goodbye each as I made my way back to the Surgical Outpatients Department which, as it happened, was almost empty now. Wow – had I been that long?!

CHAPTER THREE

The News

It wasn't long before I was called into the original consulting room by a nurse. I was told to take a seat and wait for the doctor. Then the Registrar appeared from the other doorway. He sat opposite me on the edge of the bed, his hands clasped together. He had that look...you know....like he's about to say something serious yet sensitive in a calm fashion.....You could hear a pin drop.

"I've had a look at the sample I took earlier," he began.

"Oh yes?" I was very interested.

"You did the right thing in coming in," he added, then continued:

"I'm afraid you do have a cancer tumour which is malignant," he obviously didn't believe in beating around the bush!

"Oh," I replied. "Oh well, I suppose it was bound to be".

This response seemed to shock both him and the nurse.

"I must say you're taking this very well..." he said.

"Well, what else can I do?" I asked, "It's pretty obvious, once you've discovered one of these things, that that's more or less what it's going to be, isn't it?" was how I explained my response!

He continued:

"The other samples you have just had taken in the biopsies will be taken away and analysed. However, you apparently also have a lump just under your arm in the lymph gland area. Therefore, you will need to have a mastectomy and radiotherapy treatment..."

"Oh," I said, "OK".

"We have a lady who specialises in breast care nursing who will –"

At that moment the other door opened and in walked a well-dressed, middle-aged, fair-haired lady with a sympathetic smile on her face, who made her way directly to me. The nurse left and this lady took her place on the chair next to me. She introduced herself. Her name was Joan. She was indeed a Breast Care Nursing Specialist who would be available throughout the course of treatment and longer if necessary.

She insisted on continually reiterating how this was curable so there was nothing to worry about. I thought the frequency of her reassurance, nice as it was, a little over the top. I suppose she thought I needed it. Maybe I did but just didn't accept that at the time. I mean, I'd got it, so I just had to "get on with it."

"Well, I'm not the only one," I said, "thousands of women have this – I'm not the first and won't be the last!"

She advised me that there was also a possibility of reconstruction of the breast, which I was pleased about, even though she said this would need more surgery (which her tone implied would mean an additional, unpleasant long haul) – I didn't care about that: just give me another boob!! The Registrar left me with Joan.

"This feels like a dream, actually," I remember saying, "Hold on a moment," I pinched my left arm and continued: "No, I guess it's real! Oh well!"

I seemed to find myself rabbiting on a bit because, well, she just let me.

I suppose that was part of what she was there for - to give me a chance to "let it all out", or in my case, just to give the whole background to how I let it get to this stage and then to be pragmatic about the whole thing because, basically, after all, I considered it was my fault for not coming sooner and, ultimately, as I seemed to mention to everyone I met after this, "what can I do about it?" It was up to the hospital now. I just thanked God I'm around in this day and age when it can be detected and when there are possible solutions and treatments. If I had been born a hundred years ago, it would have been a different story!

She finally took advantage of a rare pause in my conversation to suggest I ring my husband to pick me up, even though I had arrived in my own car. But I said I preferred to drive home, even though I knew it meant a seventeen mile journey home for me after all I had been through today but I didn't want to leave my car in the street (I hadn't managed to obtain a parking space in the hospital, so it was parked a good half mile or so away in the main town thoroughfare). She asked if I wanted to speak to my husband anyway and, because I didn't have too much money left on my mobile phone, she kindly allowed me to use her office phone, the other side of the waiting area.

I followed her there, past just a couple of people seated in the waiting area. It was a small office with fairly modern furniture in it. She showed me a chair by her desk with a phone on it and I proceeded to dial, explaining as I did so that it was always hard to get through to Simon as he was working on a building site. She stood beside me, waiting. There was no reply. I wasn't surprised. I tried my home number in case he had got home early – after all, I had been at the hospital a long time (it was now 5.30 p.m.); it was quite possible he was home now.

Finally, he answered.

"Oh, hello!" I said.

She nodded, smiled and left the room, closing the door behind her.

"How'd it go?" he asked. I could tell by his tone he expected quite pleasant news. He had forever told me before I came that I "would be fine". I had to disappoint him.

"I've got cancer," I said. Then I suddenly couldn't contain myself. I burst into tears. I couldn't hold them back. I was almost annoyed with myself. I didn't expect this! I tried to explain how this conclusion had arisen and how my day went and, eventually, I managed to compose myself. I searched through my handbag with my free hand for a handkerchief and gave him a chance to respond as I wanted to blow my nose.

Actually I can't remember much of how his response went. I suppose I was too busy searching for a handkerchief. I remember he did sound surprised and disappointed at the news, though. He definitely didn't expect that result. I suddenly felt sorry for him. It wasn't the news he expected – or wanted.

I couldn't find a hankie. I told him I was originally ringing for him to pick me up but that I was OK now and would drive myself home. He said he would pick me up if I wanted him to, he didn't mind at all, but I didn't need him to. However, I told him it would be nice if he could cook something for me for dinner! There I was, thinking of food at a time like this! He agreed to cook a meal, saying that that was the least he could do (or maybe he said that later, after I thanked him for doing it – I can't remember for sure; I wasn't really myself during this phone call...)

Anyway, Joan eventually returned, with her sympathetic smile, which was appreciated a little more this time.

I thanked her for the use of the phone and confirmed that I was OK to drive myself home.

She gave me her business card and said if ever I needed to speak to her at any time about anything to give her a ring. She was one of four such nurses who would be with me all the way during this episode and even after, if required. She said the hospital would send me a letter now advising a follow-up appointment date, probably next week.

After we said goodbye I had another proper look for my hankie and finally found it. I blew my nose and then headed for the nearest ladies' toilet. I noticed the couple still seated in the surgical waiting area. I hoped they hadn't heard anything. I was embarrassed. By my phone call. By the fact I was unlucky enough to contract the Big C in the first place and hadn't been as prepared as I had initially thought. By everything.

I left the hospital. It was quiet now. It was like a Sunday. I walked past the near-empty car parks. So THIS was the best time to get a space, I thought! I braced myself for the long journey home. I would normally race down the A30 at top (legal!) speed but not this time. I had no inclination at all to drive anything over 40. I must have looked like a lost tourist! Even admiring the breath-taking scenery meant nothing to me right now. I kept trying to tune my car CD player to songs that weren't sad but even those that weren't seemed to have words that I was able to fit to my new situation, which managed to depress me. I suppose that's what most people do to relate to them. I told myself I wasn't going to cry again. I just wanted to get home and see my family. I wanted a hug. I wanted....oh, I don't know.

I looked into my rear view mirror. Cars occasionally overtook me. Well, it was rush hour, I suppose.

In a few hours I would be back along that road in the opposite direction, on my way to work. Strangely, that didn't bother me at all. The staff were great, even though they hadn't known me for very long (two weeks!).

When I finally arrived home, I couldn't wait to get in and see my other half. We hugged. I was OK.

I apologised for crying down the phone but assured him I was OK now and....actually.....I was. Then I smelt burning.

"The oven!" I cried out and raced towards it. He beat me to it and opened the door.

"Is this on 'oven'?" he asked, pointing to the circular knob at the top.

"What? No! You've got it on 'grille'!" I exclaimed.

He carefully retreived a burnt pie from the oven.

I sighed.

"I thought I had it on "oven", he said sheepishly.

I turned the dial to the correct position then smiled.

"Put it back," I said, "hopefully we've caught it in time and it's just the pastry that's burnt!"

Well...at least he tried!

CHAPTER FOUR

Then It Hit Us

The next day I was doing my usual journey to work along the A30. I was overtaking various vehicles, listening quite happily to my CD. However, the more I listened, again I found myself "welling up" and taking deep breaths in an effort to prevent it, after all, I was in charge of a fast, moving vehicle. I glanced at my rear mirror. Nothing was behind me. All the traffic was to my left in the slow lane. It was no good. I had to pull over into the slow lane also and compose myself. I told myself they would cheer me up at work. And they did.

The first question I was greeted with when I entered the office was "how did it go?" They all thought I had just gone for a regular mammogram which, of course, I had. It just turned out to be a little more than that.

"I've got it," I remarked casually as I removed my suede jacket and hung it behind the door.

You could feel their shock and sadness sear through the room. I related the events of the previous afternoon to them as concisely as possible. Alix, who had a few problems of her own, commented that I was "emotionally strong" and that I should stay that way! She asked how my family were coping, particularly my other half. I said he seemed quite OK – we just hugged in the kitchen soon after I had arrived home. She commented that, though this appeared to be his outward reaction initially, it was probably going through his mind at work today. As it turned out, she was quite perceptive.

Later in the day a Detective Sergeant gave me the telephone number of a friend of hers who had undergone what I was about to go through.

She had had a mastectomy and had now come through "the other side", very pleased with her new boobs which were now bigger than her original small size! I determined to contact her at some point, deciding it must help hearing how someone copes who has actually been through the process.

Once I was back home, I decided to ring round various friends and relatives all round the country, those closest to me at least, to inform them of my status. Why should I keep the bad news to myself?! Amongst these were the Committee Members of my own Amateur Dramatic Society which I had been instrumental in setting up the previous year. I had actually been offered a part in this year's forthcoming production, for which I had begun to learn lines, as well as my usual work preparing and organising virtually everything involved with a major production, as I was Chairperson and Founder! Jerry, the director offered to meet with me to discuss the future. We arranged a meeting at our house soon after.

That evening, I felt a little tired so went to bed earlier than usual.

The phone rang whilst Simon, my hubbie, was upstairs in our bedroom. I was already in bed, so he picked up the receiver. It was his mum. Bless her, she's rung us nearly every day since the diagnosis, i.e. a whole year. He stood beside the bed and spoke to her for a while, obviously about my situation. I noticed him occasionally wiping his nose with a handkerchief but just thought it was the beginning of a cold – he was long overdue, not having had one for ages. He eventually passed the phone to me. I had a little chat with her whilst he sat down on the bed next to me. After we finished talking I replaced the receiver and could sense something was wrong (yes, apart from my cancer I mean). He wiped his nose again with his hankie.

"Have you got a cold?" I asked. But somehow I knew the answer even before he replied.

"No," he said, stuffing the hankie into his trouser pocket. Tears started to well in his eyes. A sight I'd only ever seen once in our eighteen years of knowing each other.

Suddenly, it was like a scene from the film "Love Story":

He broke down and managed to say "I don't want to lose you..." between the sobs. My colleague had been right. Well, that was it. I leaned forward and put my arms around him, saying he wouldn't but that I needed him to be my "rock"; he had to be strong for me. "I'm not strong," he replied, but I knew different. "I've been thinking about it all day...." My colleague had been right again.

I never knew a man could love and care so much as to reveal his emotions in this way. I knew he loved me but....to miss me that much when I'm gone?

I knew I had to be the strong one in this instance but I still couldn't help but let go of a few waterworks myself at this point. I knew that farther down the road our roles would be reversed and I would rely on him like no other.

CHAPTER FIVE

Life Imitating Art

A couple of days after my hospital visit, whilst at work, I was beginning to itch terribly on my left, plastered boob, so much so that my colleagues insisted I ring my GP for an emergency appointment there and then. I eventually gave in and did so.

Despite arriving on time for my appointment, I waited over an hour to be seen. Of course, this was only once I could bear the pain no longer and finally went up to the reception asking how much longer I would have to wait. That was when my name was called!

The young, male doctor (not my own) apologised for the long delay. I explained, in a matter-of-fact fashion, the history behind my current painful discomfort.

After waiting for a female nurse to be present while he examined me, he commented to her about my very "matter-of-fact" attitude.

"Everyone keeps saying that," I said. "Well how am I supposed to react?"

The nurse explained that everyone handles it differently. I gathered that much!

The doctor then informed me that, fortunately, I had no infection and that I must just have been allergic to the large bandaging attached by plasters all around the breast.

"That's good," I said, obviously referring to the lack of infection.

The doctor then proceeded to remove the bandages and plasters and replace them with much smaller patches, much to my relief.

That evening, Jerry came round as arranged. He handed me a "Get Well" card, which I thought was nice, and we discussed how I was doing and what I wanted to do about my involvement with the group. We both agreed it would ultimately be best if I stepped down, not knowing exactly how long this could go on for, gave my role to someone else and distributed my "Chair" responsibilities amongst the other Committee members. I was choked about giving up my role, especially as he had specially given that part to me without an audition because it was "me" (I hope the other members don't read this!). After all, I had originally just wanted to act in my new hometown, not run a drama group (some have "greatness thrust upon them"!!) Ironically, the character was a fairly elderly lady who always bemoans her physical ailments, of which there were many – a part I would soon be familiar with! Talk about Life Imitating Art! The fact that I had cancer didn't seem to bother me as much as losing this role – especially as I had already started learning my lines! He suggested perhaps I still do that in case I felt able to be a stand-in! Or at least, I might be able to do the announcements at the beginning. I was happy with that. Well, as happy as I could be under the circumstances.... We agreed I would still be more than welcome to attend any rehearsals or meetings if I felt up to it. As it happened, I think the actress who took my part did a better job than me anyway, so I guess things do happen for a reason!

On Saturday of that week, a lovely big bunch of flowers in a vase arrived via Interflora from my father and brother (my mother having died seven years ago of leukemia). I was really pleased and surprised! I never usually hear very much from them unless I contact them. But obviously when I do they pull out all stops!

On that Sunday Dave, another group member, had apparently heard the news and popped round with a little bunch of orange carnations! We chatted about my situation for a little while and discussed how I wanted to proceed within the group. I related to him details of my discussion with the director. He understood, stating that, of course, my health was more important than having a role in a play.

CHAPTER SIX

Bosom Buddies

Not long after being given her mobile number, I took it upon myself to ring the DS's friend who had contracted the same illness a few years previously, and who has had the "all-clear" after seven years. She's a livewire! More upbeat than me! I found all the information she had to give very useful: "I'll tell you things the hospital won't tell you to expect!" she said. And she did.

Well, apparently (though of course everyone is different) with chemotherapy she told me I should expect:

Regular vomiting, particularly straight after each session (being supplied with anti-sickness tablets and steroids to try to prevent the same), hair loss (or thinning at the least), nose bleeds, dry throat with food having a metallic taste; oh, and one good thing: no periods! Although they may come back at the end of the entire session in a not very pleasant way. She told me to expect to be very tired after for a long time and to re-consider acting in my drama group – she suggested I get a "stand-in". She added that certain smells used to set off vomiting after chemo sessions. It took her seven years to get the "all clear".

Oh, and she also mentioned that she found herself having lots of nightmares for some reason (something else to look forward to - not!).

Regarding hair loss, she found a wig too itchy after a couple of weeks so resorted to wearing a head bandana (but with my son's cheeky sense of humour and desire for practical jokes, I don't know how I'd cope with that!). One positive thing about the hair loss was that you then don't have to shave your legs or under your arms for the duration! However, you have to draw on your eyebrows and wear false eyelashes as these probably vanish as well. Even your pubic hairs vanish! It's like being a little girl again – or a baby, as you have no head hair! Although she did add that your head hair comes back in lovely condition, just like a baby's. But the weird thing is that it usually returns in a totally different colour and style! For instance, she was originally a long-haired, straight-haired blonde but her hair came back short dark and curly! Well, I said, Simon could probably do with a different woman by now! After all, we'd been married 17 years – he might end up with a blonde or redhead! My hair was dark brown at this point and had got a natural "kink" in it anyway so there was no telling what style or texture it would return in. Mind you, my grandparents, uncle and brother all have/had auburn hair so...we'll just wait and see...

Also, with her mastectomy and lymph gland removal, particularly the latter, she was left with a numbness in her arm pit and her arm. To combat this, she had to wear a plastic sleeve (and this arm became bigger than her other arm) and is unable to lift anything more than 10lb with that arm. In fact, one is not supposed to do any heavy lifting of any sort, eg, shopping – EVER! Also, the numbness makes shaving under her arm more than tricky – there's no way to tell if she's cut herself because she can't feel anything! Plus, your immune system goes. There was also a possibility one could contract a condition called "Lymphodema" – something to do with the filtering of lymph fluid which prevents infection.

Regarding reconstructive surgery, she explained that they "move the flesh around from behind to join up onto the new breast and they don't use your old nipple – they concoct a new one!"

(On speaking to another friend at a later date, she informed me that a new nipple is actually "tattooed" onto the breast! She also added that an after-effect of radiotherapy – apart from extreme tiredness and needing to use a lot of cream because it was like severe sunburn – is a permanent tatoo on your chest where it's done. I envisaged the like of "Love/Hate" or "I Love Mum", but she explained it was just a tiny black dot and actually showed me hers.) I later discovered there were other ways to reconstruct one's breast, by using tissue from the stomach (qv later chapter).

My other friend was very clearly pleased with her new breast; apparently she used to be an "A" cup but was now a "C"! (I'm currently a "D", but surely they make the new breast the same size as the existing one?) She added that she knows at least four people who all had it done and all are fine.

She commented about how I should expect up and down moods throughout. There would be tearful times, happy/pragmatic times, etc. She added that she just had to stop buying some newspapers that forever seemed to be reporting something about cancer! She found it too depressing. I soon found out what she meant!

She told me to make a list of questions to ask the Consultants at the hospital before meetings. She also advised me of the Patient Advice Liaison Service (PALS) if I needed more information.

One positive thing, she added, was that both myself and my spouse would be entitled to six free massages each at the Force Cancer Support Centre!

We arranged to keep in touch and perhaps meet some time if I feel up to it.

CHAPTER SEVEN

Keeping Abreast of the Situation

Every day a few more "Get Well" cards arrived for me. In time, I had more of these than I normally get for my birthday! They included one signed by all the drama group and even one signed by everyone at my previous job – a law firm – brought round personally by Zoe, a friend of mine (a conveyancing solicitor from the same firm). She stayed for a while and we had a chat over a cup of tea about things generally, apart from my health, for instance how things were with the firm now and my successors.

She asked how my sixteen-year-old son was taking the news. I related to her a brief conversation we had had just that evening:

We were seated together on the sofa watching TV. I happened to remark about how I used to notice people's ears once I had had mine pierced, and now find myself looking at women's boobs.

"Why?" he asked, obviously a little perturbed.

"Because at least they've still got theirs," I replied.

"Well, you'll still have your...." he glanced at my chest "....one" and continued nonchalantly watching the television.

It's funny but I did find myself frequently commenting, especially to the ladies at work who occasionally bemoaned various aspects of their social lives, that at least they had their breasts! And even their hair!

My son found the whole situation quite intriguing. Soon after hearing the news, particularly about the forthcoming mastectomy, he confronted me in the kitchen with his arms stretched out in front of him and his hands cupped together, stating:

"Just imagine, mum – after the surgery, the surgeon will be standing by the edge of your bed saying 'Look - this is your boob!' "

I couldn't help but laugh before giving an obligatory frown, stating that that wouldn't quite be how it would happen!

Clearly everyone reacts to news in different ways. Fortunately, I appear to be surrounded by a section of society with, possibly, a warped sense of humour, which I found interesting to say the least! For instance, on telling my own brother that I would obviously have to go to hospital to have the operation, he advised me not to read any long books. (To anyone else I know that must sound appalling but as I too must have a warped sense of humour, I did find this amusing.) My best friend from school also advised the same but I told her I prefer to write rather than read, to which she replied "Well, don't write any long plays!"

I did stop writing a play I was working on but only to give me time to write this book. (I just hope I get to the end – I don't want anyone else finishing it!)

Myself, every time I have a shower with my shower cap on, I cover my eyebrows with both my index fingers to see how I would look without hair there! How l survived those six months I don't know. Although, when I was first diagnosed, I consigned myself to just imagining I wasn't going to hospital – I was merely going to stay in a hotel where they also happen to do cosmetic surgery on your breasts which is purely for aesthetic reasons, not cancer – after all, so many women do that when there are no health reasons! Also, whenever I can (usually when I'm at least semi-naked!) I cover my hand over my left breast (the one I won't have too much longer) just to see what it will look like. I even showed Simon once, trying to encourage him to get used to the idea. It's just so unfortunate, as I tell many others, that he happens to be a "boob" man! Why couldn't he be a "leg" man? Just my luck! Oh well, I tried to console myself by thinking that it's not a "functioning" part of my body – I'm not having any more babies – and it's not my eyes, so I can still see the lovely scenery around the area I've just moved to, and it's not my hands, so I can still type my plays, etc.! It's not my legs so I won't need to go around in a wheelchair. I'm actually quite lucky – after all, my hair will grow back (so everyone keeps telling me) and boobs can be reconstructed or at least replaced with a prosthetic piece for insertion into your bra.

Something I found strange was that, after being diagnosed initially, I had no desire to have any alcohol. Now wouldn't you think someone might take to the bottle on being given such news? Maybe I just didn't realise quite how serious it was, I don't know. But considering how much I like the odd glass of Baileys, for instance, I suddenly found myself not only not drinking it for the first week or two, but not even *wanting* to drink it, or any other alcoholic drink.

As if being told the news I had cancer wasn't enough, I found myself empathising with other victims of the illness. Everywhere I looked, every page of a newspaper or magazine I turned, every programme on TV or even commercials, there was some reference to it. And everyone I spoke to had either had it or knew someone who has had it. It was far more prevalent than I had ever realised. Even though I knew my own father contracted it some time ago and, to this day, is still having regular check-ups in Hertfordshire, I still didn't realise just how many people have connections to other sufferers.

Unfortunately, cancer wasn't my only worry. Having only just been at my new job in Special Branch for a couple of weeks, I volunteered to leave due to the unknown prognosis, as it didn't seem fair for them to train me only for me to have to leave soon afterwards. I thought it would give them a chance to train somebody else for the job as soon as possible. Of course, this now means we have only one set of wages coming into our household now. And with our only son soon to leave school, even my Child Benefit payment was soon to cease. Simon didn't earn anywhere near as much as he used to when we lived in the south-east of England. Pay levels are much lower in the south-west - as are jobs! Especially with a recession looming.

The following Tuesday I had an appointment with my Consultant Surgeon – the boss of the Registrar whose name I couldn't remember!

Simon came with me. We waited the usual hour in the waiting room – made worse by the fact that it seemed that everyone else waiting was passing the time by reading magazines which all happened to be open on pages with headings like:

"My Freaky Boob!" or "I want a boob job!"

I couldn't believe it! Didn't they know the primary reason for patients awaiting consultation in this area?! Strangely, in a way, I found it quite amusing before it eventually got on my tits!

The waiting area gradually became more and more empty until finally I was called. Luckily, just before Simon fell asleep, as he does in these situations! (He's no company on plane and train journeys, where sleep prevails!) He accompanied me to a different room to the one I had been in the previous week.

I was a little perturbed to be asked to put on another of those little gowns again but I dutifully obliged whilst my spouse waited in another section of the curtained-off consulting room.

A tall, handsome, brown-haired, suited gentleman (though not as handsome as Simon of course – maybe just a little bit taller!) came through. He introduced himself as Mr Ferguson, Consultant Surgeon, and shook my hand. He was accompanied by Sandra, another Breast Care Nursing Specialist – a dark-haired, younger woman than Joan.

He briefly examined my breasts (I was starting to get used to being groped by strangers now!!). Strangely, despite his good looks, I was able to disassociate myself from the man doing such a thing to my body. It's as if your body "switches off" when it's in a "business" situation! He then told me to get dressed.

I then joined them in the other part of the room –Mr Ferguson on his side of the desk, with Simon and Sandra on the other. I sat between Simon and Sandra.

Mr Ferguson had my file in front of him and looked quite business-like. As he started to speak I told him to wait a moment as I pulled my chair forward towards the desk, straightened myself up and took a deep breath, preparing myself for whatever news he had.

"OK, go ahead", I said, ready for the worst which, as far as I was aware, I had already been apprised of by his registrar. How much worse could it get? Maybe his confirmation would make it sound like there was no going back...

He gave me then what I thought was wonderful news – he told me that I didn't appear to need a mastectomy ("appear" being the operative word, I later discovered). Well, that was it! I exuberantly interrupted him stating that I couldn't hear anything else he said because that, in itself, was so great!

I couldn't contain myself – I turned to Simon and cried out "You see – there IS a God!" Simon smiled warmly.

He went on to explain that I would still need radiotherapy, though, as well as chemotherapy, tablets, surgery, CT scan (which I later discovered stood for "computerised tomography". Just thought I'd mention that, to make up for my lack of expertise with other medical terminology!), bone scan and blood tests (not much then!) I was so thrilled about keeping my breast that I just didn't care about the rest! Wow! However, I was a little perturbed by my Consultant advising me that there was still a one in five chance that I *may* need a mastectomy in the future, depending on these test results.

I mentioned about the little three-day break we intended having in a few weeks and he asked if I wanted to start treatment before or after that, to which we decided to have the surgery first then our break before the main treatment. He was going away himself soon, so he popped out to get his diary. Meantime, Sandra asked if I had any questions and said she would give me their booklet with a lot of information about the treament after this meeting (some booklet – gives "War and Peace" a run for its money!)

Mr Ferguson came back and we all agreed on a date – a date that will go down in "infamy"! 2nd May was the date for my lumpectomy and lymph gland removal from under my left arm. I was (cautiously) ecstatic but felt emotionally drained.

I learned that there was only one cancer lump in the breast and the other one was in the lymph glands and, as yet, no mastectomy was required (famous last words), <u>but</u>, he again emphasised I would still need blood tests, CT scan and bone scan in the next two weeks to determine if the cancer had spread. Then I would have my operation on 2nd May (1¼ hours), probably returning home two days later on the Sunday. This would be followed by radiotherapy for two weeks, then chemotherapy, then special tablets (tabiofloxim or something!) for after the chemo. *(I obviously misheard his description of the medication – what he actually must have said was 'Tamoxifen'!)*

I would be able to drive a couple of weeks after the lumpectomy so we could go on our planned mini-break to North Devon on 16th May. I was told I would receive a letter confirming the date of the operation.

That Friday was my last day at work. The next day I drove Nick to the Powderham Castle Horse Trials where Simon was working. It was a rainy day. The turf was soft and yucky! I spoke briefly to Simon who was setting up the jumps after the horses and riders did their stints, including Zara Phillips. However, after a slippery stroll through the mud around the various equestrian marquees and tents, I decided to head the twenty miles back home, leaving Nick to help out the team and myself to adjust to my new situation......

CHAPTER EIGHT

No News Is Good News

The following Monday it was time to pick up Toby's "designer" boot for his cancerous/arthritic front left paw. It was black and silver with laces (yes, laces!) and cost £10. It looked really cool. The only problem was it was too big for him really and flopped about an inch over the edge of his paw when he tried to walk. Needless to say it didn't last long! We still have it in the house somewhere I think. Anyone want a designer pooch boot?

23/4/08: By chance, I saw advertised on SKY TV a film called "My Breast" – a true American film based on a real woman's experience around fifteen years ago. I toyed with the idea of watching it. Should I or shouldn't I? Oh, what the hell! I couldn't resist. As it happened, it was an interesting film. I related to some of it, as was inevitable I suppose. The lady in question found herself taking particular notice of women's hair (or lack of it) – especially those who were already going through chemo – and was clearly terrified of the future, as was I. However, I found it interesting that she had a decision to make regarding whether or not to have a mastectomy, as I was under the impression that we don't really have that choice over here. Well, not if we want to survive apparently! The only real choice seems to be to try to live or to die. In the end, it turned out that she didn't need one after all. I felt her relief!

27/4/08: I read in the Daily Mail about more new treatment for breast cancer being tested, i.e. blood tests, long before the first signs of even a lump. However, just my luck: if the results prove positive, this treatment won't be available for another year. Good news for future sufferers I suppose.

It also mentioned that the latest super bug to hit hospitals is C.Diff, which is apparently worse than MRSA (Methycillin Resistant Staphylococus Aureous? – I tried to learn the phrase when I was the Administrator of a Mental Health Home).

As if that wasn't enough, it added that breast cancer, though being the cancer with the highest success rate, is also the biggest female cancer with 500,000 women dying worldwide a year.   So....no wonder my Bosom Buddie stopped reading that National newspaper!

CHAPTER NINE

And so it begins....

22/4/08 : This was the date I returned to hospital for a CT scan. Simon took me. I didn't have too long to wait before being shown into a very "futuristic"-looking room! I remember thinking it was like something from a sci-fi movie! The centrepiece was a very large piece of metal equipment: A bed was protruding through a high, wide arch. I was told that, during the process, some patients have spoken of an overwhelming desire to urinate! <u>What?!</u> Well, fortunately, I had only just visited the loo, so I hoped I would be able to convince myself at that time that it was only psychological! Actually, that's just what happened! It was indeed a strange feeling, after lying down on the bed which slowly moved under the arch before pausing. The nurse was in a room partitioned off from my area (she was the lucky one!). I could hear her voice being transmitted through speakers embedded on the inner arch near my head as I lay, virtually helpless, under the arch, with an overwhelming feeling to visit the loo again! She instructed me to hold my breath a few times before the bed slowly moved back to its original position. Well, that was it. The whole process didn't take long at all so I departed and Simon drove me back home.

The next day, whilst shopping at our local supermarket, I bashed into Kelly, a young colleague from my last job but one: the local solicitors. We both had a love of amateur dramatics and, indeed, I had cast her in the panto I had written for the company for their previous Christmas social event! We had a brief chat – she asked how I was and wished me well, before we both continued shopping.

On the 24th I decided to go to my hairdresser, Frankie, and ask her to cut off my fairly long, thick, dark locks, in preparation for losing my hair during chemotherapy. She was shocked at the news of the cancer but kindly obliged and offered to also help at a later date with doing my hair – even styling any wigs I may have – this was appreciated.

The following day I went to see my GP to sign me off work. That evening Zoe called round for a chat.

28/4/08: Whilst in town lunchtime, I decided to pop into said solicitors to say hello and met Ann, the receptionist, and my friend. We chatted a little while about my condition, etc. before I eventually bid them farewell.

The next day, Alix from the Police Force, with whom I had the most contact there, rang me at home to see how I was doing, I thought that was very nice of her, especially considering I no longer worked there. I informed her that I had a "Pre-Op Assessment" at the hospital to look forward to the next day (30th).

The next evening, the plumber came round to give us a quote for fixing a new boiler – we hadn't had hot water or central heating for a good few months....everything goes wrong at the same time, doesn't it? Something about "it never rains but it pours"?.....

So came the day of my Pre-op Assessment. I had arranged to meet my "bosom buddie" after the assessment but, as it turned out, she had to cancel due to a "review" at her work.

Anyhow, on the day of the assessment, after arriving on time for my 9.20 am appointment, I had a half-hour wait in a long corridor, along with other patients. After a while, my height and weight were measured, then I was shown into a small room where I was asked a lot of questions for completion on a form by a nurse. Then I was asked for a urine sample after having my blood pressure taken. Before this, however, I was told I should be tested for MRSA. She informed me that this was done by way of swabs up my nose and at the back of my throat. This entailed a very long, chopstick-style stick with a type of cotton bud on one end being stuck up one nostril. However, because the stick was so long I had trouble locating my nostril and found myself giggling somewhat! I was waving it around the general nose area but just couldn't quite find the target! The nurse had to assist. Then she gave me another one which I thought was for the other nostril and managed to insert it into the vacant nostril, whilst laughing – I felt so silly with two long sticks protruding from my nose, even more so when I caught a glimpse of myself in the mirror by her desk! Apparently I was laughing so much that the female doctor had to enter the room to investigate the noise – I don't suppose they get many patients laughing their heads off in hospital! Then it was explained to me that the other swab was actually to take a sample from my throat! Hmmm....talk about embarrassing!

Eventually, the doctor took me to another room and gave me a general check-up (chest, back, etc.) then I was told to go along to other departments for a blood test and ECG and return with the results – which no-one passed on to me...

8am Friday 2nd May: This was "D-Day" for me – or the first of many, as it turned out. Simon drove me to hospital for my lumpectomy op – surgery to my left breast and also the removal of the tumour from the lymph gland nodes. There was no bed available on my arrival so we had to sit and wait in the waiting area immediately outside the ward and in front of the reception area, with a lot of human "traffic" moving through and around the area. After waiting a few hours, I was apologetically told that I would have to get changed into a gown in the toilet next to reception, as they were still awaiting a bed for me!

The anaesthetist had to discuss forthcoming events with me in the corridor and a nurse clipped a shiny white cardboard bracelet onto my wrist which stated my name, date of birth and hospital number. She also clipped a green one onto my wrist. When I asked what that one was for, she explained it was to show I had an allergy.

"What allergy?" I asked.

"Your sickness with anaesthetics," came the reply.

Then I was told to go into the next room – a small office – where I met up with Sandra, the Breast Care Nursing Specialist whom I had encountered on my meeting with the Consultant Surgeon. Soon after a brief chat with her the Registrar entered and drew on me. That is to say, he drew a large arrow on me just above my left breast, obviously leaving nothing to chance! Then he proceeded to clue me in on what was going to happen, e.g. I would have two incisions made and they would remove the tissue from around the lump and lymph glands. I may also still need more surgery; possibly even a mastectomy at a later date. This did not please me. I seemed to keep getting conflicting information – one minute I'm overjoyed at not needing to lose a breast, the next I'm trying to psychologically prepare myself for one of the worst operations a woman can have! Anyway, some time later I left Simon in the waiting area with my luggage as I was accompanied to the operating area by nurses and Mr Ferguson, the Consultant Surgeon. Having no bed to wheel me in on (which I was a little disappointed about), I just walked to the theatre with them. I took the opportunity to ask Mr Ferguson about the results of my CT scan, to which he replied that it revealed my liver, kidneys, etc. were all OK. Well, at least that was something.

Not remembering anything about the operation (fortunately!), I found myself waking up in Recovery, where I had an oxygen mask on. They apparently now had a bed for me and once I was in the ward, they replaced the mask and put a tube into my nostrils which fed oxygen into me – I had often seen these in medical programmes on TV and, call me ignorant, but I never really knew what they were! I was also on a drip and beside me in the bed was a blood drainage bag, attached by tube to my left breast.

Later, Mr Ferguson came to see me, informing me that the op. had been successful. They removed what they wanted and I should stay a couple of nights – going home thereafter if I felt up to it. There would be a meeting to discuss the results Wednesday week. I remarked to him that, believe it or not, this was the best op I had ever had! Simply because I wasn't vomiting! (I usually vomit after an operation – allergic reaction to general anaesthetic, apparently) He replied that this was because I had told everyone beforehand about my sickness history. I had no pain now.

My fellow patients on the ward weren't so lucky, pain-wise; one lady had had a gall stone operation and was still in agony, another elderly lady had painful shins where she had fallen (before the op presumably) plus a young patient had had the same as me except that she had had a blue die inserted, which made her urine and tears blue! Freaky! Also, it meant her breast would remain blue for a year – even more freaky! She and I got on quite well, especially as we had similar problems! I felt particularly sorry for the "gall stone" lady, though – a fairly attractive, slim lady in the bed next to mine; apparently her husband wasn't really up to scratch. It seemed he liked his drink a lot, as well as socialising – well, he was quite well off – had his own company and large house. I think he did visit at least once while I was there though.

It took a while to take a peak down my dressing gown at my boob. When I tentatively attempted this, I was a little surprised that it didn't look as mishapen as I had expected, even though it was covered in bandages. However, a little while later I went to the bathroom, which was the other side of the corridor, near the reception. As soon as I entered I noticed a large spider dangling in the toilet! I tried to ignore it and decided to just take a better look at my chest area. I carefully manoeuvred the hospital gown so as to reveal this. I had a clearer, fuller view now. I moved my left arm out of the way which revealed that ny left breast had a good third of it missing – the side of it was sort of "indented". My face dropped. I re-dressed that area quickly and returned to the ward.

Simon and Nick visited later. I had a good bed but the button you had to press to raise the back wasn't operating and I wanted to sit up. Nick had a great time pressing all the buttons ("trying to assist", so he said) and it did eventually work. However, when I was in an upright position, that meant I could no longer reach my locker!

I was hungry. Dinner was clearly being served shortly after 6 pm but there was no meal for me. I had to wait an hour after everyone else had had their meals (chosen the previous day) before I was given what was left over! I heard the elderly patient opposite complaining about her meal; clearly, she wasn't "all there" as she moaned: "This salad is too cold!" The nurse had to explain that that was the nature of salad!

I was awoken at midnight by the lights being switched on in the ward. A new patient was being wheeled in. The nurses were trying to be quiet but to no avail. Once they were back in the reception area immediately outside the ward, I couldn't sleep for them laughing (at least they were enjoying their work), tapping away at the keys on the computers, dropping things, stapling, closing doors – it was amazing how aware I was of even the slightest noise which one wouldn't ordinarily hear amongst the hustle and bustle of daytime life!

Then, to cap it all, the elderly patient, kept trying to "escape"! Her efforts were hampered by her being attached to a drip unit and catheter, but this didn't stop her attempts at trying to reach the doors at the other end of the ward which, she didn't realise, only led to another ward! She kept calling out that she believed the staff wanted only to shoot the old people and gas them, because she read about it. The poor staff spent most of the night trying to usher her back into bed every time she got out! Needless to say, I had little sleep that night.

3/5/08: My left arm started twinging below the middle. I decided to put up with it.

4/5/08: I had a blood test. Later my left arm started hurting even more. I realised, at one point, that my armpit was quite numb. There was no way to tell whether or not any deodorant I may spray there was hitting the spot! I could feel nothing. You could tickle me there and I wouldn't laugh! I might frown though.

During my stay a physiotherapist gave me a leaflet explaining the exercises I needed to carry out with my left arm. I was told my armpit would remain numb for a while but at least I had no need for a special "sleeve" for my arm, which apparently lots of patients require after this op. I was informed that I shouldn't lift anything heavy (so pick yourself up Simon!), especially with my left arm, for quite a while (eg more than 10 lbs in weight) and I would be receiving daily visits from a District Nurse in order to, primarily, keep an eye on the drainage bag.

I found out for myself just how hard it was to even raise my arm just a little. Plus, the first time I tried to raise myself to sit up in bed, I couldn't put any pressure on my left arm, hand or wrist to facilitate the action; I struggled to raise myself, using only the right arm, and lean back against a vertical pillow.

Two days later I felt well enough to go home, although trying to get dressed was a nightmare! The drainage bag, still attached to my breast, hindered the "dressing operation"! However, I finally managed to remove my hospital gown and put my day clothes on before Simon and Nick came to pick me up.

The elderly patient in the bed next to mine noticed my "chauffeur" – my handsome husband! – gathering up my belongings for me, and remarked: "You've got a good-looking one there!" which cheered me up (and no doubt Simon!).

We bid farewell to them all and left for home.

I received my first visit from a District Nurse the next morning to adjust the drain.

She also came the next day, when I also had a visit from one of our friends, Christine, who is a dairy farmer's wife. She brought round some drinks and we chatted for a while. She told me her son, David, and his wife Tabitha were expecting a baby girl soon, making four grandchildren for her! She kindly offered to take me to hospital if ever I needed a lift and Simon wasn't available.

So far, I had received 16 "Get Well" cards, all neatly displayed around the lounge.

As I was now unemployed, with no financial 'sickness' or 'unemployment benefit'. I therefore had to apply for other state benefits to help me live now. I had many....MANY....forms to complete in order to get some kind of financial relief to help pay bills, prescription charges, transport costs, etc. (But that's another story...I may regale you with it later if you really want to be bored)

Whilst taking a very brief walk to the local post box a few yards away (in order to post these MANY forms), I remember looking at the lovely scenery surrounding our street, at the hills and trees in the distance, and thinking, even though I've got a potentially life-threatening illness, I could still appreciate the warmth, fresh air and scenery. I couldn't walk very fast – any vibration to my upper body caused some pain in the breast area – but just those few moments breathing in the fresh air and observing the environment I was fortunate enough to live in, gave me something of a "lift" before I returned to our semi, where I then had to sit down for a while to "recover" from the brief exercise!

From 6th – 8th May we had a "mini-heatwave" when I sat mostly in the garden (not realising this was to be about the best weather during the whole of 2008!) On the 8th it was very breezy (see – it changed already!). I remember wondering how on earth birds and flies stay on course in such weather! I was sitting in our patio area, overlooking our small pond which was surrounded, in part, by various plants and bushes. I noticed some frogs leaping around there, then I decided to feed the fish. Toby stood beside me, watching – as he does whenever there's any hint of food around! I sat down again and stroked him. I was just too tired to take him for a walk (He doesn't walk anyway – he always runs!)

Bed-times were a nightmare. Every time I wanted to turn over I had to physically "cup" my left breast in my hand in order to help it turn with me, whilst, at the same time, manoeuvring the drainage bag attached by a very long tube to my breast (hopefully without squashing it!)! One night, I awoke to discover the bag had fallen out of the bed and was lying on the floor, still attached to me via the tube! My efforts to retrieve it unfortunately woke Simon, who was not amused!

Simon had to help do the cooking. Once, I forgot about not using my left arm for heavy weights and tried to open the oven door with my left hand. I had no idea an oven door was so heavy! I immediately had to change hands, the weight was too great!

Wednesday 7th May: the District Nurse I was expecting failed to turn up so I rang the hospital who had originally arranged all the visits, who told me to ring the doctor's surgery. When I did, I found myself talking to Mally, a friend of mine from my drama group – she works at the surgery! She promised to get someone round asap and that afternoon the District Nurse did turn up. She said she would remove the drain the next day (recommended by the registrar) due to the risk of infection. She said the Breast Care Nurses at the hospital would contact me for results on a date sooner than 14th May. The District Nurse gave me her telephone number to call, should I leak once the drain was out.

On the 8th my breast suddenly swelled up like a balloon – much bigger than when the tumour was inside. It prompted fears of it bursting and leaking! The District Nurse removed the drain when she visited. The tube she pulled from my breast was much longer than I expected (I never watched it going in, so I didn't really have any idea of its length)!

The next day my breast was so uncomfortable and "tight", as well as being slightly red and huge, that Simon had to drive me to hospital to see if they could release some of the fluid inside it which was causing the growth. I said if the same thing happens after the mastectomy, that would be great – from no boob to a sudden big one! But then they'd have to increase the size of the other one else I'd be lop-sided! Maybe someone should invent a bra for two different sized breasts! Talk about breast enhancement! I could see the headlines now: "Cancer causes unexpected Boob Job!"

Unfortunately, the Water Board chose this particular time to do some major job that involved a lot of road works around the city which, naturally, led to a lot of diversions around the hospital. This, in turn, added an extra five miles to our already long journey. Oh joy!

The hospital staff successfully drained some, or rather a lot(!) of liquid from my breast. The relief was almost identical to when I was breast feeding my son and he took all the milk from me!

The following day found me having to surreptitiously hold my left breast whenever I ran upstairs, or even if I was a car passenger and was being driven over bumps – the "sleeping policeman" kind, or just potholes! I wasn't able, at that time, to drive myself.

.

CHAPTER TEN

A lot of bull...

I had 18 "Get Well" cards now!

13/5/08: Nick was away on a school trip – a river cruise followed by a barbeque. I had the day to myself.

I had a visit, this time, from TWO district nurses, one being a trainee. I was interested to learn that the other one had previously had a similar operation to mine.

The day passed as it usually did, with me struggling not to lift anything heavy, whilst also being careful to support my left breast if I manoeuvred myself too fast at any time!

Unusually, Simon didn't come home till late – VERY late! Like 1.50 a.m. instead of 6 pm! (having started work at 6 a.m.!) The reason? Well, apparently, during his working stint at the Devon County Showground, a bull that was due to be shown at the show had managed to get loose from his pen and was creating havoc, eluding capture by running off into various fields in the area! Everyone was chasing it in an effort to get it back; they even tried using a tractor to steer it in the right direction. It literally took them many hours to retrieve it – eventually doing so by nearly two o'clock the next morning! Fortunately I was able to get in touch with him to find out what was going on. I didn't get to sleep until he was home. Oh well...at least it took my mind off my breast! (notice I said "breast", rather than "cancer"...my mind was rarely on the cause of all my health problems, rather the treatment.) Since then, on relating this incident to various friends, I notice it is usually met with a raised eyebrow and a look as if to say "Well, that's what he *tells* you is the reason he was late...! Hmmm...

14/5/08: I had a hospital appointment at 4.05 pm, to be given an update on my results: apparently, I did need a mastectomy. So I had to get my mind around that scenario again; preparing myself psychologically

16/5/08: Simon, Nick and I all headed for our weekend break at a Horse Farm in North Devon. Toby came too (limping along!) We arrived in the afternoon and had a great time. We rambled through the fields, seeing various animals: horses, cows, sheep, etc., observed their own shire horses pulling buggies around the area, visited the local tank museum, took lots of photos (I tend to do that a lot!). I even got chatting to a friend of the other visitors who informed me that she, in fact, went through the same procedures as I was going through/would be going through and, when I mentioned that I wasn't really allowed to drink, she said she took no notice of that advice herself and drank lots every day! I decided not to take too much notice of that and continued to be tea total – at least for a while! The wife of the owner of the farm commented that I was in for a long haul (that didn't do anything to cheer me up!). Anyway, the "getaway" made for a nice break – I knew it would probably be my last "holiday" for quite some time (and I was right).

19/5/08: I arrived for my pre-arranged visit to see my Oncologist. The appointment was for 3.40 p.m. I eventually got seen at 4.20 p.m.! (I later learned that they apparently book everyone in at the same time so it's usually "first come, first served".)

Joan, the Breast Care Nurse I saw at the initial diagnosis, was also in attendance. It was like attending an interview...all very formal. Dr Goodman, the doctor, was a middle-aged man with a moustache, wearing dark-rimmed spectacles and a bow tie (plus other things of course!). He basically wanted to know that I understood the procedures Mr Ferguson had informed me I was going to experience, i.e. chemotherapy, the operation, radiotherapy, reconstructive surgery. I was told I could see photos depicting the different stages (I was keen on that – really!). I had to sign a consent form regarding these procedures.

He gave me further information, such as I may never get my periods back (oh, joy! No more stomach cramps!), but still needed protection for sex for a while after treatment. I needed a thermometer (which we have) to check my temperature and I was to ring the hospital if ever I was ill during chemo – as that would mean that I may have an infection, in which case I would need to be in hospital for approximately four days and, in the worse instance, may even die if I was unlucky (yes: that would be unlucky....)

He said some patients like to know the risk factors/life expectancy involved regarding whether or not they had treatment and asked if I wanted to know about mine. I said yes. He put various details about me (age, non-smoker, etc.) on his computer. Joan moved out of the way so I could sit next to him to get a clearer picture. After a while the results of my projected life expectancy appeared and he printed a copy for me. They showed that, in my condition, 72% of patients would live if they had no treatment whereas 89% of patients survive if they had treatment. Naturally, I therefore opted to have treatment!

They checked on my breast, which was getting swollen again, so the nurse made an appointment for me to go in again for drainage the next day at 5.30 pm. I also got a prescription for tablets for the pain – very strong ones, called Diclofenac, to combat the intense pain.

CHAPTER ELEVEN

Getting it off your chest.

20/5/08 – 5.30 pm: Simon took me to hospital for the breast drainage. After waiting for 45 minutes, we were the last ones left in the waiting room. Simon actually fell asleep to the point that he began snoring! (he gets bored very easily). I remarked to the admin woman near reception that we <u>must</u> be next now! She laughed (in a nice way). Then I was called into a side room. I woke Simon up and he accompanied me to the room. They drained 450mls of liquid out of my breast – 4 trays! I felt an overwhelming feeling of relief and comfort on the left side of my chest.

We went home. I had 23 "Get Well" cards now!

The next day I felt extremely grateful and, indeed, humbled by being granted a loan for a boiler by the Macmillan's charity. Up till now our heating and hot water system was up the spout – bad timing especially if you're ill. I was fed up with constantly having to take the kettle full of hot water up to the bathroom for a wash then forgetting to bring it back to the kitchen when I fancied a cup of tea! To say nothing about being cold in the house without heating, barring an electric fire.

The following day I read the leaflet supplied to me by the hospital regarding all the effects/side-effects of having chemotherapy. I got the very definite impression that my body was going to be out of whack in two weeks! I was already on tablets since the operation.

I bought myself a silver SOS talisman from a local jewellers shop, to wear on a chain around my neck. It stored details about my name, address and blood group, etc. It also would advise medical people not to take blood pressure or do injections on my left arm – forever. The talisman itself served a double purpose in that it also concealed the permanent sunburn marks I have just above my cleavage!

A couple of days later my boob begain growing, as usual; I was becoming accustomed to the scenario: let it grow, drain it, let it grow, drain it!

I rang Irene, an old friend from my previous drama group. She had moved house at a similar time to ourselves 18 months ago, but was now living in Surrey. She didn't mind me using her to "get things off my chest"!

We also bemoaned the current oil crisis of the time which was causing massive petrol price inreases. I moaned about having to do a 40 mile round trip to hospital on a regular basis to drain my breast, then we discussed the latest terrorist explosion to take place in the country – a nail bomb in the county city, let off by a 22 year old Islamic convert. To lighten the conversation, my friend apprised me of a possibly little known fact: that there used to be a legendary race of warrior women called Amazons, who used to cut off a breast (their own) in order to be a better shot with a bow and arrow – she said I was on my way to being one of them! (She actually sent me a "Get Well" card depicting such information in cartoon form!)

I read my horoscope (for Libra) in the Daily Mail on 24/5/08 – it said "Where there's life there's hope and where there's a will, there's a way." Hmmm....

That Saturday we all attended a "birthday barbecue" at Brian's (Simon's boss) farm, which we all enjoyed. I thought it might take my mind off my health but, alas, I found myself discussing my situation with the guests, who all sympathised with me, relating their own experiences to me. I was told about a young boy of only 3 who had it and of a friend of theirs who went about life as normal, for instance running and organising all kinds of events – cancer didn't hold her back!

We drove back home around 10.30 that night and I was musing over the evening's events. I suddenly piped up to Simon:

"I should be OK, having had that alcohol now, shouldn't I? I mean, I haven't had my tablets since one o'clock. It won't affect my breast will it?"

"Of course not," he replied, "It's going to come off anyway."

I pondered on his words and said, somewhat pensively, "It's.....going to come off.....anyway...."

"Not on it's own!" he reassured me!

I remembered a quote by an actress on the television soon after. It was a comedy programme. Something hadn't turned out quite right in the scene and she remarked "Well...life is full of new experiences..." I equated that to my situation, it was so true.

Whilst discussing my soon-to-be lack of hair during chemo, Nick commented that I will "look hard" when my hair first starts to re-appear – I would look like a skinhead instead of a "slap-head"! How's that for a new experience?!

28/5/08: Christine drove me to hospital for my regular "breast draining session"! The surgeon's registrar did the job. Whilst there (in the hospital, not the cubicle where I was being drained), we saw her mother-in-law, who was in a different ward. She had recently suffered a stroke and was barely talking.

I was given more tablets by the nurse to help with the pain, etc: paracetamol, Diclofenac enteric coated tablet (50mg) to be taken three times a day, anti-biotics: clinamycin capsules (150mg) (2 to be taken four times a day) and Flucloxacillin (try pronouncing that!) capsules (500mg) (one to be taken four times a day). They also gave me Zipiclone (3.75 mg) sleeping tablets as I was having difficulty sleeping because of my breast! I must have really rattled with all those inside me! I was really fed up "popping pills" and completing long, extensive forms in order to survive financially (when I heard, at the outset, that cancer was expensive, I couldn't understand that....I can now.)

53

I suddenly realised at one point that both my surgeon and my oncologist had names of electrical appliances! (Ferguson and Goodman!)

One evening, I was watching a programme on TV called "99 Bizarre Surgeons Blunders" (not the most sensible thing to do at that time, I know). They revealed a case (in America fortunately!) of a woman who underwent a *double* mastectomy. However, somewhere in the process her notes got mixed up and, apparently, it turned out that she didn't have cancer at all. Poor woman. Another case was about a patient whose surgeon operated on the wrong eye while she was awake but, because of paralysis due to the anaesthetic, she was unable to stop them removing the wrong eye. I watched the show in disbelief then looked down at my breast, fingers crossed!

The weekend of 30th May my family and I attended our mutual friends' (Brenda and Alan) 25th wedding anniversary in Berkshire, together with my in-laws. It was a garden party. Whilst there, I acquired not one but two gnat bites – one on each foot - fortunately not on my arm, on which it was ill-advised to have any kind of "injection"! (I managed to keep it under wraps with a cardie, so the gnats obviously went for my exposed feet instead!) I remembered the Queen a few years back calling one year an "annus horribilus" and thought, "Yep – this one's my annus horribilus"!

We also visited some old friends Cliff and Kathy, whilst in the area (we discussed the eventual radiotherapy treatment and tattoos!) before taking the long drive (2 ½ hours) home.

CHAPTER TWELVE

Another Hurdle

2/6/08: Wirh my chemotherapy due very soon, our kindly neighbours, George and Barbara, loaned me five books to read from their extensive book shelves during the treatment. I remarked that it was like a library service and asked if I needed a card, to which Barbara replied "No – and we won't even fine you if they're returned late!" She was very sympathetic and commented to George: "I don't know how she can be so upbeat about it."

I set her straight and retorted: "You wait till next week when I'll be like a vomiting zombie!" How right I was!

The same day I had the plumbers in to start to fit the new boiler and replace an old radiator in the bedroom (everything happens at once, doesn't it?) They had to do a lot of drilling and removing/installing pipework from under the lounge floor into the kitchen. At one point they had to cut off the water (so there was no chance of a cup of tea!), then I discovered the electricity had been cut off (barring the lights). However, apparently, I only needed to put the trip switch on, which I did.

Between the noise of the drilling I managed to catch a glimpse of a TV comedy show, which just happened to be about a man's parents discussing death and funeral arrangements, before another programme set in a hospital. Then I read on the internet that Senator Edward H Kennedy was having brain tumour surgery, chemo and radiotherapy! Well, I couldn't cope with that! Why was I continually being confronted with situations that reminded me of mine?!

By the end of the afternoon the plumber had to give me bad news (OK, not as bad as being told I had cancer!). He said he couldn't finish the boiler that day due to the gas pipes' positioning, plus Simon would need to fill in the wall for the flue from the new boiler to go through, as a smaller gap was needed.

"Oh," I replied, "Wanna biscuit?" I continued eating the one in my hand, whilst my other hand was holding a biscuit tin.

He just laughed and couldn't believe I seemed only interested in food!

The next afternoon, I was given a lift to hospital by Christine, who accompanied me to a "wig fitting session" at the Force Cancer Support unit of the hospital. It was either here or a trip to the city at a special store that catered for this (Dangles or Dingles or something like that!). I chose Force, mainly because I knew it and it was nearer. This was also the building where we were given free massage sessions (my husband and I)! It was like a mini-hotel: a little winding path bordered by plants and trees led you to the entrance inside of which was a lounge-type reception, filled with comfy sofas and armchairs, coffee tables, books and magazines, even a birthday card stand for cards to be purchased, proceeds of which went to the charity. There was a little library room off the lounge which also had a corridor leading to the massage rooms, the wig fitting room and another lounge area. As soon as you arrived and explained the reason for your visit, you were offered a drink (tea, coffee, hot chocolate, not alcohol!) and biscuits. The large windows all around the perimeter of both lounges allowed you to see into the garden area outside. It was very secluded, with wooden tables and chairs and countless plants, flowers and trees all around: a very peaceful setting. All this just because you're ill!!

We were soon shown into the wig fitting room, filled with tables on which were suitcases containing lots of different wigs. It was actually good fun, sitting down in front of a mirror, trying on lots of different coloured/styled wigs. Christine took photos of me in each one to help me decide which one I would later choose. I even suggested she took one of me with the stocking-type head cover which concealed my dark hair; it made me look bald. She looked a little worried but I assured her I wanted to have a shot of it as a record of how I would look when I eventually went bald through the chemo, just to get used to the idea. She still looked worried, but took the photo anyway. At the end of the session, the pleasant wig fitter lady and myself persuaded her to try on a couple of wigs herself and I took photos of her! Eventually, I chose a medium-length, layered, chestnut-coloured wig for myself that was currently unavailable due to having only just been produced– there was a photo of it in the catalogue and I particularly liked it. It was called "Gina" – they all had girls names! I was informed that it was more expensive than all the others, which were approximately £120 each, and therefore required me to pay £20 – the £120 was provided by the NHS – I couldn't believe it!

At another "fluid draining session" re. my boob, Joan, the Breast Care Nurse, asked how the wig fitting session went and I replied exuberantly "Great! I can't wait to go bald now – all the wigs were so nice! Better than my own hair!"

She asked, somewhat concerned, if I was always a "jokey person" to which I replied that I was – I wasn't trying to hide any fear or anything....I just find humour in everything! I can't help it! I told her that I was writing a book about the whole experience and she said that was probably good therapy. I said that if it was, that was only a by-product because, actually, I had to stop writing a play in order to do this and, primarily, it was to encourage any reader not to do what I did – that is, wait too long before diagnosis – in order to avoid what I was going through now!

The following morning I had the first of many, many blood tests, taken at my local surgery on the outskirts of town. This was apparently the required procedure before every session of chemotherapy treatment.

That afternoon I had to take my car to our local garage due a problem with one of my tyres getting hot (more expense!). I can't remember what the cause was but I remember they managed to sort it out, which was a relief as I needed my car more than ever now, with my hospital treatment.

5/6/08: I attended hospital (again!) for my "Pre-chemo Chat". I arrived at 1.30 for my 1.45 appointment and was offered coffee and biscuits, a jigsaw and magazines to read! I was taken to a side room in which stood a TV set and a couple of seats. A nurse sat opposite me (I think her name was Alison) and told me what to expect regarding the chemo, including, during the initial stages, red urine! (This was due to the compound of the chemicals put into my system in the first few months – the dreaded "Epirubicin", which I've doubtless spelt incorrectly!)

I told her about the recent gnat bite I had acquired and asked if it was still advisable to go ahead with the chemo, especially as my left arm was also hurting and my breast was swollen! She found a doctor who examined my arm and breast and said they wouldn't affect my treatment. They both laughed sympathetically about how I kept trying to get out of the treatment! Alison advised that I watch a video about chemotherapy but that I should not bother to watch the video immediately after it, about radiotherapy. Naturally, when the time came, I couldn't resist seeing at least a little of the one about radiotherapy but, after a small bout of guilt, decided to switch it off. The chemo tape showed a variety of patients; some of whom had various problems with side-effects, particularly vomiting, while others said they had no problems at all! I knew my situation would more likely be akin to the patients experiencing side effects!

Well....that was it. I went home and tried on a bandana for the first time to get an idea of how I would look with hair loss during the treatment. I had previously been told by a nurse in the Oncology department that it was more than likely that I would experience this due to the first chemicals being Epirubicin, which was very strong (the last three months of the six-month treatment would be CMF chemicals: less potent and severe but more frequent in application).

After reading some leaflets, I discovered that, apparently, it was better not to wear any silk scarves on my head when I was bald as these would just slide off my head! Other material was better. Luckily I had a variety of scarves to choose from that I had bought in the eighties. I rarely throw anything away – just ask Simon! In fact, I have a little notice up on the kitchen wall which I bought in Canada some years ago (the notice, not the wall). It reads 'the greatest way to find a use for something is to throw it away'. How true, I thought! On a later visit to the Force centre, I purchased a nice, blue velvent turban, with space around the edge in which to fit a thin scarf to ring the changes: this helped me to co-ordinate my outfits!

I tried, as best I could, to prepare psychologically for the forthcoming treatment. Little did I know that how I was feeling at the moment would be the best I would feel for at least six months.......

CHAPTER THIRTEEN

"D-Day", 6th of June...the Real Fight

I couldn't help but liken the onslaught of my chemotherapy to being taken to the electric chair for execution!

Simon took me for the first treatment. We barely managed to get a parking space. The cost of parking for anyone having this treatment was, fortunately, reduced!

We waited in a nice, large lounge area, complete with lots of armchairs, a comfortable blue sofa, coffee tables, magazines, books, birthday card stand, a large tin of chocolates on one of the tables (yummy!), even a large fish tank similar to the one at my doctor's surgery! The tables had unfinished jigsaw puzzles on them. Not being any good at jigsaws except the very large ones for toddlers, I declined to try to finish them.

At the entrance to the lounge we were greeted by a representative from the Force unit who offered to make us tea or coffee together with biscuits, which was totally unexpected and very nice indeed! I donated some money in the appropriate tin and appreciated the refreshment.

Simon waited with me on the sofa. A secretary was busy typing away at the large desk in the corner. I was slightly apprehensive about what was to come. Simon did his best to put me at ease, telling me it was for a good cause. Yeah, OK.

Eventually a male nurse called Vince appeared in the doorway and showed us into a side room next to the two large treatment rooms. Inside was a bed, table, sink and what looked like a very tall table lamp standing on the floor! I learned this was the "ice cap" for patients to wear if they wanted to reduce the risk of hair loss, which I wanted to do. However, he explained that the effect would be greatly lessened due to the particular first chemicals I was to have and Simon, on putting his hand inside the cap attached to the top of the stand, warned me that it was exceedingly cold. We thought that, if that was how it felt on a hand, we could only imagine with fright just how exceedingly cold it would be on a head....especially if worn for an hour or so, as required! To make things worse, I was informed that I would have to wash my hair first and go under it with a wet head of hair! Well, that was it! Needless to say I changed my mind about that part of treatment – especially as it wasn't essential!

So he showed me into one of the treatment rooms: a very large room, with about twelve upright, comfy chairs in it and two beds at the end. Most of them had "drip stands" and monitors beside them and a few of them were occupied, both by men and women – some of whom were wearing bandanas on their heads, most of whom were engrossed in reading books or drinking tea whilst attached to the equipment via thin white tubes on their hands, which didn't seem to bother anyone.

I sat on the chair nearest the door; Simon sat next to me, putting my handbag on the floor beside him (oblivious to how it affected his macho image!). I was told to put my hand in a bowl of quite hot water – something to do with showing up my veins (that is, making them appear, not embarrassing them). Then Vincent inserted a canula into the top of my right hand, attaching me to the drip-feed, in order to facilitate insertion of saline and the red-coloured Epirubiscin in a syringe. My hand was getting cold as it seeped into my body, so he gave me a nice warm blanket to put around it to maintain heat, then gave me saline again. Three more syringe-fulls of the Epirubiscin were given in total and an hour later, before I left, he supplied me with three lots of anti-sickness tablets with a name that sounded like something mentioned on the film "Star Wars" (metaclorian?!).

We left the hospital at 12.15. I had a white bandage covering the insertion wound on my hand. Despite being slightly tired (a fact I had been informed about by many people prior to the event), on the way we stopped off at a local supermarket. I didn't feel too bad at that point though and, in fact, remember thinking that it wasn't as bad an ordeal as I thought it would be! Little did I know....

I checked my emails on my return and it was nice to see Don, a committee member of my local writing group, expressing concern and a wish to visit me some time. We arranged a date for this (24/6).

Four hours later I felt nauseous and took a couple of the tablets the nurse had given me earlier. However, they didn't help as I soon began vomiting thereafter, violently, consistently, until the 10th (four days later). It caused me to be bed-bound and lose a lot of energy, as well as weight (something good came out of it then – no need to diet!). I noticed my skin began to get dry and spotty, then I needed to use a mouth wash to try to combat the mouth ulcers I was getting. I also had a stomach ache and was tired and generally lethargic: I found it hard to concentrate for long periods at a time, especially when it came to reading, writing or even just watching television and talking on the phone.

11/6/08:   Christine called in with a huge, lovely bunch of pink Peony flowers picked from their farm garden. They lived in a large, rambling dairy farm which doubled as a bed and breakfast hotel, in the midst of a lovely valley, surrounded by picturesque hills. Her husband, Alan, was actually born in the very large, old house there, which was built in the 14th century. It was full of nooks and crannies (or crooks and nannies?). Some of the floors sloped from one end to the other, making you feel a little sea- sick if you weren't used to them! A lot of the interior doors were quite wide and were made of very thick wood (don't ask me what type). We actually got to know Alan and Christine simply by being guests of theirs several years ago. They were such an hospitable, friendly couple and the area was so lovely where they lived, it enticed us to move over a hundred miles away to share in the joy. We didn't just move for the sake of it though – we wanted to move anyway but couldn't think where.

Once, before we moved, we brought Simon's parents, George and Cynthia, with us to stay at their farm. It was Cynthia's birthday and

Christine made a lovely birthday cake for her! Now how many B&B hostesses do that?

Nick used to help Alan milk the cows and even drive the tractor occasionally. Simon sometimes helped Alan chop the fire wood and I (very occasionally!) assisted Christine in the kitchen.

Back to the Peonies. Christine and I chatted for a while. Another friend, a member of my drama group, called in to see me. However, it turned out that her visit to me followed one of her own to her GP. She had discovered a lump in her breast and I could tell she was a little unnerved and distraught. "Oh dear," I said sympathetically and rose from my seat on the sofa, "I think we'd better give each other a hug!" I sat next to her and we hugged.

I tried to calm her down, explaining that that didn't necessarily mean she had the same as me, and even if it did, I tried to make light of the various procedures involved, at least the ones I was going through. I told her that, anyway, having discovered hers earlier, it would probably be much easier to cure than mine and she probably wouldn't need to go through everything I was going through. I hoped that made her feel better but somehow I didn't really get that impression.

13/6/08:   Simon and I had free massage appointments at the Force Cancer Support Unit. Simon opted for a back massage and I went for an Indian Head massage. The massage therapist commented, whilst doing my head, that I had nice, thick hair. "Not for much longer," I replied and settled down to listen to the music while she massaged my head.

CHAPTER FOURTEEN

The Rocky Road

14/6/08:   My lips started to feel sore so I put some lip salve on them.

I decided to check if I had received any emails but discovered I had THIRTY-FOUR to catch up on - all because I wasn't able to check on them regularly due to feeling tired all the time. Naturally, reading and replying to all these gave me a bad headache!

Soon after every chemo session Simon kindly brought me a cup of tea in bed every morning, which duly exited via my mouth soon afterwards. Because he was then at work the rest of the day and I was usually bed-bound with weakness due to constant vomiting, I relied on Nick to bring me up my lunch – usually soup – which, again, duly exited my mouth almost immediately, but it was nice while it lasted (the soup, not the vomiting).

At 8am on the 15th, Simon went to the local hall to help my drama group's backstage crew set up the scenery for our forthcoming play, a comedy. As it was Father's Day, at 6pm he, Nick and André, a young friend of ours with whom Simon used to work, went fishing down at the coast. They didn't catch anything except, maybe, a cold. Oh, but Nick did catch a sock and Simon and André caught seaweed and a bit of the sea bed!

16/6/08:   Two members of my drama group, Dave and Jenny, popped in to see me (Dave with his Jack Russell who, unfortunately, didn't take very well to Toby!) After he left, I arranged, with Jenny, to have a day out when I was feeling better, perhaps to the seaside, and have a coffee. She gave me some encouraging comments, such as she thought I'm a "fighter" (I assumed she was referring to my fight with cancer!).

17/6/08:   I had 28 "Get Well" cards now!

Christine and I had lunch at tea rooms in a nearby village, before she kindly drove me to hospital to pick up the wig I had ordered. Whilst there, we also visited her mother-in-law in one of the wards. She was still quite poorly and was barely able to speak a word. I noticed how similar she was, in looks, to her son – there was no mistaking they were related!

I wore the wig home. Simon had just arrived and was standing by our back gate as I was dropped off. He had a silly grin on his face. I therefore knew to expect a silly remark and, sure enough, one came out of his mouth:

"You look like Dusty Springfield!" he taunted.

"No I don't!" I took umbrage. Just because the style was quite "bouffanty" on top of the head in a layered fashion, I could see no resemblance myself.

On the 18th and 19th I had workmen in to sort out the new boiler and do electrics for our new shower. At 2.20 on the 19th I had an appointment at my Consultant Oncologist's clinic at the hospital. He was actually away on leave so I had to be seen by another doctor. Whilst waiting in the usual waiting area for the usual considerable period, I got chatting to a couple of other patients – a husband and his wife – who were trying to do a crossword. The husband asked me "What do you call a tightrope walker?"

I replied: "Stupid?"

He said it began with an F, so I answered: "Flipping stupid?" Well, I was bored!

(Apparently the answer was something like "Funumbulist".)

I was eventually called to see the doctor. She informed me that the previous, second blood test had revealed that my liver "number" was high – it was apparently 21 before and was now 116 – whatever that meant. She thought it was quite possibly a mistake but it needed to be double-checked after I had a Hickman line inserted on the 25th. (This was a tube to be fed into my chest, near my heart, to facilitate insertion of chemicals and withdrawal of blood for tests, to save keep having injections which would apparently not do me much good in the long run.) If the liver number was correct, I would need liver ultrasound (whatever that is). Hmmm.....

We discussed my severe vomiting since having chemo, to which she recommended that I take what are apparently called "Zombie" tablets. I couldn't help but let out a laugh. I stuck my arms out in front of me, waving them around, zombie-fashion, and said "Will they make me walk around like a zombie, then?"

The doctor smiled and informed me that, in fact, patients have commented that they do actually make you feel like a zombie because they are the strongest anti-sickness tablets around so, therefore, cause extreme tiredness.

We discussed other side-effects, like my hair loss, which wasn't apparent yet, and she told me to just wash and brush my hair very gently (which I was already doing!) I mentioned that I was having watery eyes and always awoke in the morning with them stuck together! This was due to the chemo, I was told – as was everything apparently! Any problem – just blame chemo!

20/6/08: 12 – 1pm: Two husband and wife friends of mine, Irene and John, from my previous drama group in Berkshire, were passing through on their way back from Spain, so they popped in for a chat. They brought me two nice bunches of freesias!

5 – 8pm: Zoe came in for a chat. Then, in the evening, newly married husband and wife André and Claire called in to see us (I was certainly

getting popular!). Nick was attending one of his friend's party in a local village. It took place in a large marquee tent. Nick asked if he could stay out till 11 pm. I remarked that his return times were getting later and later, to which – quick as a flash – he replied: "Well I'm getting older and older!"

22/6/08:   8 am: Simon was picked up to help finish setting up the scenery at the hall again. He got back around 4 pm. (a bit of useless information for you there.....)

24/6/08:   I had 29 "Get Well" cards now!   (More useless information!)

Between 2 and 4pm I attended a "Look Good, Feel Good" session at Force. Together with about twelve other women (a variety of ages, some of whom wore bandanas), I sat at a very large, rectangular shaped table, on which were placed a lot of mirrors and various objects to do with makeup. There were a few "instructors" (presumably from commercial make-up companies) who were on hand to help show us how to apply make up properly. They gave each of us large white simulated leather make up bags containing make up that was specifically tailored to our own complexions, as well as expensive perfume (to make us "feel good"!) There were 18 products in all – at a total costs of approximately £2-300 each – given to us free! I couldn't believe it! I'd never been so pampered! We all left looking and feeling like a million dollars!

5.40pm: Two committee members of the local Writers' Group (Treasurer Don and 92-year-old Secretary Joan), called round to see me. They gave me a lovely bunch of flowers, as well as a box of Belgian chocolates and a special pen with the group's name on it! In order not to feel left out of the group due to my illness, they asked if I would be well enough to judge a forthcoming writing competition that Autumn, as I was unable to contribute by writing. I was flattered and informed them that I had actually stopped work on my own play because of my extreme tiredness, but if I felt able, I would be delighted to judge the competition.

That evening Simon and I had a meal at our local pub/restaurant, only a few yards from where we live.

At 2 pm the next day I arrived at the hospital to learn about a minor operation to have what is known as a "Hickman Line" inserted about a centimetre away from my heart (to facilitate the chemo treatment and blood tests). During my visit I encountered the couple who were doing a crossword in the other waiting room recently, plus – talk about a small world – one of Nick's young school teachers, who was awaiting the same operation! We all sat watching a TV in a very small waiting room adjacent some wards; I think the film was "Sinbad"! The sound was down low. At one point, someone suggested we play "I Spy" (no, not me) because we seemed to be waiting quite a long time! A lady eventually popped in, asking if anyone wanted a cup of tea, just as a nurse appeared, calling my name to be seen! "Oh, I don't believe it!" I moaned, but the nurse said I could still have my tea (and I did!).

I was taken through a ward and into a treatment room at the end of it where I was measured, weighed and had yet another blood test, answering a few questions put to me by a male nurse (whether I had allergies, etc.). A doctor entered soon after to explain the operating procedure to me, accompanied by a large drawing depicting my chest area and the directions of the tube and "cuff" – a larger part of the tube to prevent it coming out of me! I had to sign a form giving my consent to have the operation performed and my understanding of the various risks involved, not least of which was "dying"!

CHAPTER FIFTEEN

A Hair Raising Experience- Hair Today, Gone Tomorrow!

26/6/08: I awoke very early in the morning to find a disturbing sight on the pillow: a few strands and clumps of hair staring back at me. So it had begun...my long awaited and long dreaded "hair loss"...

I had a very early appointment – eight o'clock in the morning - to have my Hickman Line inserted at the hospital. Simon said it was akin to me being like one of the "Borg" aliens on Star Trek – I likened it to being like an android! I was actuallly the first patient to arrive at the ward and was led to another, very modern and quiet ward for treatment. Simon was with me as usual. We had to wait for more staff to arrive before I was eventually asked to swop my clothes for a long gown. I was quite impressed with this gown – it actually preserved one's dignity in that it wrapped over itself around your back – hiding everything! (Not like the old types of years ago.) I had to remove my earrings and rings, except my wedding ring, over which the nurse put a plaster. The nurse also placed on my wrist a white paper bracelet with my name and hospital number on it. She asked me the usual questions in order to complete yet another form. When asked if I had good hearing, I couldn't resist responding with "Pardon?!" Fortunately, she laughed. She asked if I had eaten anything prior to coming in. I said no, as that was what the doctor had advised the previous day. However, the nurse – in agreement with another one in the ward – was surprised and said I could have had at least a cup of tea because I was only going to be under a local anaesthetic! I was stunned as well as thirsty!

Simon and I sat on chairs situated between the long reception desk and three or four beds. I left him in charge of my belongings, as usual, and he was quite content to sit and read a magazine. Although, had he known how long he was going to end up sitting there, content isn't quite the word I would use!

After a while I was put on a trolley bed and wheeled along a lot of corridors, with an accompanying nurse, to the special theatre. Unfortunately, there was a bit of a wait when we arrived and they had to leave me in a kind of "reception/waiting room/corridor" area, next to a wall near an open area full of cabinets and a wall clock staring back at me. There was a fair bit of through traffic (doctors and nurses) but at least there were a few paintings on the wall to admire to pass the time, including a montage right next to my bed, which had obviously been created by children.

After a while, a nurse came up to me to ask me a few questions....the usual, you know; name, address, allergies, etc. (You'd think they would have known all the answers by now!) She took a note of the hospital number on my wrist band, apologised for the delay – due to a staff meeting, no less, which was due to end around ten a.m. I believed her. It was about 9.30 at that time! They produced another blanket for me for extra warmth.

Shortly after this I could hear another trolley bed being wheeled up behind me. I thought I recognised the voice of the patient. I let her answer the doctor's questions and waited for him to disappear before I twisted myself around to see her.

"Hello!" I cried, "I thought I recognised that voice!"

It was Nick's teacher.

I warned her about the wait due to the meeting, so she suggested we play "I Spy"! So we did!

A doctor came up to me during this and apologised for the delay before vanishing again!

Ten o'clock came and went. I was eventually wheeled around the corner into the operating theatre. A large operating table stood in the middle, surrounding by all sorts of medical/technical-looking machinery, albeit not as weird as the CT scanner. There was a monitor directly in front of the operating table. There were a few medical staff in the room, as well as a few seated behind windows in an "observatory" room high above, to the left of the room.

I was lifted onto the operating table and then the surgeon introduced himself, holding a lot of papers in his hand, and started to ask me to sign a consent form, to which I replied that I already had the previous day!

His female assistant, dressed in requisite gown and cap, proceeded to adjust my gown, whilst maintaining my dignity, to enable the surgeon to do his job. A local anaesthetic was applied by the surgeon. I tried to observe the procedure on the screen in front of me but his assistant told me to turn my head on its side, facing her, covering the side of it facing the surgeon so I couldn't really see anything other than her. I remember talking a lot – I couldn't help it. Maybe it was just to take my mind of him inserting a needle into my chest followed by a long, white tube.

The operation didn't take long really. I was soon being wheeled back to the ward to an anxious Simon.

"Where have you been?" he asked.

I explained the wait I had had in the corridor due to a staff meeting!

I was wheeled to the corner of the ward in readiness to have my second chemo session. I asked Simon to buy me a cup of soup and some crisps as I was quite hungry by now. Whilst he was gone, a nurse began chatting to me and we found out we both originally came from the same part of the country – London! But we both preferred it here in the countryside!

Whilst partaking of my refreshment a little while later, another nurse approached me in readiness to do the chemo and I asked if it was alright to carry on eating. She said it was. Thus she began attaching the syringes to my new Hickman Line to the "bung" at the end of my newly inserted tube. I can't say too much about the procedure because I still feel sick just writing about it! Anyway, needless to say, after a short while, the treatment was over and I was ready to be driven home by Simon (the medical profession doesn't advise patients driving home immediately after such a session.)

29/6/08:   I had 31 "Get Well" cards now!

I noticed I was becoming slightly more emotional since my second course of chemo treatment had been due and taken: I found myself becoming inexplicably sad just at poignant ads on the television, showing other people with cancer and the charity work. One day I even departed from my normal even-tempered manner in the local supermarket and had a go at another customer who was slighting me to her friend after I struggled to get past her trolley which was in the way. Not like me at all! I can count on one hand how many times I've lost my temper in all of my fifty years! I have a very long "fuse"...it's just that...well, at the very end of it...watch out!

30/6/08:   The strands of hair on my head (as opposed to that on my pillow every morning) were now in untidy "blobs" and clusters. I was loathe to brush it too heartily for fear of large chunks coming away with the brush. I suppose I was just trying to delay the inevitable but in vain, as it happened. The next day, after being constantly nagged by Nick to do so, I allowed him to cut my hair in the bathroom.

"You're enjoying this, aren't you?" I commented.

"Yeah, it's well cool!" he replied exuberantly.

I tentatively took my first look in a hand-held mirror before having a proper look in the large mirror on the wall. I wasn't as upset as I thought I would be; probably because I was fed up picking increasingly larger lumps of hair off my clothes and pillow, with the remaining locks getting more and more tangled and loose on my head. Somehow, being bald seemed a little easier to manage and I did have headgear to cover it. In fact, I found it quite fascinating to examine, the first time it was revealed!

Nick patted me on my newly-shaved head after he had finished shaving it;

"There you are, Slaphead! Actually, you don't look much different.."

I didn't understand how he could say that.

"Oh yes? I'm bald but "don't look much different"...?" I looked in my mirror and saw my new reflection gazing back at me; "Actually, you're right – I <u>don't</u> look much different – I just look like a man!"

I just resolved to try to avoid being near mirrors from now on! When I demonstrated wearing my new turban to Nick, he commented:

"It looks like a Genie cap!"

3/7/08: 10.15 The District Nurse attended me at home to flush my Hickman Line.

Later, I was watching a science fiction programme on TV called 'Stargate Atlantis' with Nick, specifically an episode regarding microscopic robots in a girl's body, called nanites. The scientists were using them to help cure her cancer.

"I wish I had them," I remarked, to which Nick replied:

"Well, I've got some Mecanno upstairs! I could put a few bits together for you.....!"

4/7/08: Nick's friend Alex came to stay for a long weekend. Zoe popped in around 6pm for a girlie chat.

The next day, Nick and Alex went dinghy sailing on the nearby river. I'm always a little apprehensive when he does these activities. Did

Alex know what he was in for? The last time Nick went with his gang of friends in their dinghies, half of them fell out in the river (it was a rainy day) and, as they were being swept away by the current, they tried to latch onto overhanging tree branches which subsequently fell off with their weight! One even lost his trainer shoe. Another one of them (who was separated from the rest), on seeing the floating shoe, was horrified at the thought of his friend having met with a watery end until he discovered otherwise. They also lost some of their oars so, once they had managed to retrieve their dinghies (don't ask how), they had to use "arm power" to continue their rowing! They all returned to our house, carrying soggy dinghies on their shoulders, looking like drowned rats! Oh, but this was all great fun according to Nick – it would have been boring if they just mooched about in their dinghies on a calm river!

6/7/08: Nick and Alex had a more sedate day out at an adventure park. (At least they didn't come home wet!) They stayed overnight at one of Nick's friends.

The next day Nick took Alex for a spin on his quadbike at the farm (so they could get muddy instead of wet!). It put me in mind of the time when Nick, Simon and I went on holiday to a farm in Mid-Devon a few years before. Nick had his quad with him. After having showers, Simon and I had had a massage each by the lady owner of the farm (she was a massage therapist, before you say anything!). It was then that Nick decided to convince me to take a pillion ride on his quad with him around the long, winding farm track. Foolishly, I agreed. At first it was quite good fun. He was a good, if fast, driver, cleverly negotiating the twists and turns of the track, but forgetting to warn me about oncoming, low tree branches, the twigs of which didn't fail to tap and scratch my helmet every few yards! We'd also had a fair bit of rain hitherto, creating muddy terrain, which constantly splashed up, making its mark on my legs and bottom! We eventually arrived at a four-foot high, wooden gate. He stopped the quad and discovered it was locked. He said we would have to turn back. I was not amused. However, this being Nick, he was only joking and managed to open the creaky gate. We zoomed off again down the track for another mile leading back to the farmhouse. Simon met us on our arrival, laughing when he saw me covered in mud. I thought it was just on my back and around my nether regions but, on further investigation in a mirror, I noticed my whole face was covered in muddy spots – presumably from lowering my face whilst ducking to avoid oncoming branches, consequently facing the surge of mud! So, of course, I needed another shower! Thanks Nick! Needless to say, I wished Alex good luck in his quad venture with Nick!

8/7/08: Alex took the train home.

It was this day that I discovered that Nick apparently had a girlfriend (and he's had a few, but he doesn't like to boast!). I wasn't surprised – she was always ringing him!

I was gradually getting used to my bald head (amazingly!).

9/7/08: Started to wear my new "Gina" wig to get used to it, but generally only when I went out of the house, otherwise I wore my genie cap – I mean, pretty turban! Simon tried it on once; he looked weird! I just had to take a photo!

I remember mentioning to Simon the order of future treatments:

Mastectomy, radiotherapy, hormone therapy, then he added:

"psychotherapy"!

Despite feeling continually drowsy through taking the "Zombie" tablets, I decided to pop into the local hall to see how my drama group's rehearsal was going. I was welcomed with "open arms", so to speak! That cheered me up! And I was very pleased with the progress they were making – they certainly didn't really seem to need me (a load off my mind!).

CHAPTER SIXTEEN

The Show Must Go On!

10/7/08:   The cheerful District Nurse came again to flush my line and change the "bung" on the end.

I now studied my bald head with a kind of fascination, rather than glance at it with horror!

Seeing me getting out of my car on the drive, Margaret, one of our neighbours mentioned that her husband, John, thought I looked like Gina Llollobrigida, the film actress from the sixties, in my new wig; it looked so real! I informed her that, ironically, that's actually the wig's name! She remarked that it's similar to my own hair and thought the chestnut colour was lovely!

That weekend Simon's parents visited us. We had a meal at our local Inn in the evening.

The next day, we joined in lunchtime birthday celebrations for Christine at a posh hotel/restaurant a few miles into the sticks. It was amidst lovely surroundings – trees, fishing lakes, fields. There were 13 of us all told, mostly her relatives. It was such a nice place Simon and I vowed to go again some time (and we did – on my 50th birthday in October that year!)

14/7/08:   Simon and I attended Force for our massages in the morning. When I removed my wig to facilitate the massage using aromatherapy chemicals, my massage therapist (as they like to be called!) commented that I had a nice shaped head! Apparently they see a lot of bald heads on cancer patients, so they're used to the sight!

That afternoon I took my car to the local garage for it's MOT which, fortunately, (good news) it passed! It was also due for a service some time this month but I didn't know if I would ever be able to get around to that, let alone considering the cost, as I was no longer in employment due to my treatment.

Two days later, Christine invited me to attend the local WI for cream teas etc. She drove me and a couple of her other friends, Jill and Ann, to one of the member's nice little bungalow. However, as it turned out, we were the first to arrive not because we were punctual but because we had got the time of attendance wrong! At least we had a choice of where to sit in her lovely garden! Ann unfortunately came a cropper on the deck chair she chose to sit on, as it started to collapse almost as soon as she sat on it, enveloping her in its metal legs and material! We couldn't help but laugh out loud at the spectacle – Ann didn't seem any the worse for the unfortunate incident.

Other members eventually turned up half an hour later and, though I felt rather tired, I managed to hold down a conversation or two with the other ladies and even won a raffle prize! I chose a box of Thornton's Chocolates. Unfortunately, it looked like either I was sad, or else had a cold, because I was forever wiping my nose: I don't know how many tissues I used! However, this was only due to one of the side effects of my chemo treatment – it gave me a runny nose; like sickness wasn't enough!

Later that day, I discovered Simon shaking and very hot. He complained of his joints aching. It transpired, the next day, that he had contracted gastroenteritis. Unfortunately, this was also the day of my drama group's dress and technical rehearsal at the hall. I dearly wanted to attend this as I had missed out on so much this year, which had been made all the harder because I used to do everything! I was in a quandary. Clearly, Simon wasn't well and I felt I should have stayed with him. I was torn. He just wanted to sleep and said I should go because there was nothing I could do for him. All I could do was bathe his forehead to cool him down and offer paracetamol, but he really wanted to sleep. I eventually did go, with his agreement, to the rehearsal for a little while. I explained I could only stay a little while because of Simon's ill-health.

I took a lot of photos and gave a "pep" talk at the end to the ensemble. I was very pleased with what I had seen and just gave one or two extra pointers to those assembled, but I was quite proud of my little group!

Nick went out with his latest girlfriend that day.

The next day I had to go the hospital clinic again for my usual visit to the Oncologist, or rather one of his junior doctors. I had the usual obligatory pre-chemo blood test (to check red and white blood cell counts as well as other things like liver etc.). One of the nurses rang me before I went to advise me to arrive an hour or so later due to the clinic being very busy (so what was new?).

18/7/08:   Due to Simon's illness being very infectious, I was unable to have today's chemo. The hospital rearranged the booking for the following Monday. As it happened, all this was a blessing in disguise, as it therefore meant that I was able to attend my drama group's performance on Saturday. Nick did the videoing, as he usually does for my drama groups, and fortunately, Simon was now feeling well enough to attend and accompany us. Apparently, we had sold 70 tickets for Friday's performance, which was great news for us, especially as it was only the group's second production! I managed to have a word with the Town Mayor after the performance, who said he enjoyed the performance very much, adding that he thought it was funny! (It was meant to be, of course!)

Before the performance, the group all had a Chinese meal together at the hall – although I wasn't very hungry. Whilst there I gave the group's secretary a card regarding her forthcoming visit to the hospital to check out her breast lump. It showed a fountain on the front and inside I wrote "Our ops are just little splashes in our fountains of life!"

One of our members said she knew of a lady who could give me a lift to hospital the following Monday for my third chemo treatment, which I was pleased about (the lift, not the chemo!). However, her charge was £1 per mile, which was quite hefty considering it was nearly 20 miles away! I only had £15 on me as I needed the other £7.10 for my prescription but she said that was OK.

In the chemo ward, another female patient was celebrating her 60th birthday by passing round to everyone a box of chocolates – this was well received by all! I was also given a turkey and ham sandwich by the nurse who was wheeling the food trolley round at midday. This was some consolation for sitting through the awful treatment!

I also had to have another ECG and then the stitches were removed from my Hickman Line.

My "lift" was very accommodating. She simply did a bit of shopping in the hospital shops then sat down in the large waiting room doing a crossword whilst waiting for me. She was very patient (she needed to be!).

After she got me home, I had to ring the doctor's surgery to postpone the District Nurse's visit and then eat before my next major "vomiting" bout!

The next day I had a bit of cheery news – André and Claire had had a baby girl! That took my mind of being ill at least for a little while....at least some family was having joy!

25/7/08:   I now had 35 "Get Well" cards!

Nick went on a trip for the weekend in another part of the country, via the Youth Service. It was a kind of "music festival", a wrist band souvenir of which he and his friends kept on their wrists for ever to see who could wear them the longest!

26/7/08:   I had now lost almost a stone in weight (some good news then but I suppose there are better ways to lose it!).

Unfortunately, due to excessive vomiting, I was unable to attend two barbecues that day: one held in the early afternoon in almost "luxurious" surroundings by the local Lord of the Manor and the other, held early evening, generously organised by a committee member, Dave, of our drama group and his wife Mally, at their nice bungalow residence nearby. I had been a participant of the former barbecue in previous years so my disappointment was only slight there, however, I was particularly disappointed to miss my drama group's BBQ as it was the first of its kind by our newly formed group. And I could have done with putting on a bit of weight now!

27/7/08: I was still vomiting slightly but now had mouth ulcers again, as before, and trying to eat was a nightmare - OW! The Difflam mouthwash the hospital had given me was only of marginal assistance.

One curious thing that occurred during the weeks where I vomited excessively: I found myself in dire need of extremely cold food, particularly ice lollies and ice cubes, as well as cold, creamy yoghurts – although the treatment forbad "pro-biotic" yoghurts. I also dreamed of things like diving into huge swimming pools and waterfalls, in fact, any kind of water. The thought of standing in a rain storm or a perpetual shower that never stopped filled me with a kind of relief. I just seemed to always be wanting anything cold and wet, such was the extent of the consistent passage of regurgitated food flowing out of my throat! Make of that what you will! At least I wasn't having the foretold nightmares!

Simon began giving me a new nickname: "Little Morph" because of my bald head!

28/7/08: Eating an orange was agony! It felt as if a layer of skin had been peeled from my lips, tongue and roof of my mouth and salt poured in whenever I ate. I also couldn't open my mouth really wide so eating anything quite large – for example, peaches or hamburgers – was quite tricky! And any dental visits were certainly out of the question! Yawning was very awkward too, so I tried to keep away from people who bored me (not many, fortunately!)

29/7/08: Got 36 cards now! (Okay, so four of them were all from my in-laws! They like to keep in touch – for which I'm very grateful!)

31/7/08: 11.30: Two District Nurses visited me to flush my

line. They were always very nice and chatty. I related to them the health situation of our dog Toby, saying that he had cancer of the paw before me – not that I had cancer of the paw! One of the nurses was flabbergasted to learn I was wearing a wig (I decided to wear that instead of my velvet turban that day).

3 am, Sunday, 3rd August: my Hickman line got caught in the bed. I was half asleep and kept fiddling with the tube to straighten it, whilst manoeuvering my position. I pulled it so hard that I suddenly fell out of bed! Unfortunately, there's not much room between the edge of the bed and our chest of drawers – I was sandwiched between them! This naturally woke Simon up and I reached out my arm asking for help to be raised back into bed. He grudgingly obliged!

Simon took me to the coast (later that day!) – a little town about twelve miles away where we had lunch and went on the amusements. I now have an idea of what it's like to be elderly, as I had to forever ensure I was fairly near some kind of seating and didn't have to walk far, as I got tired very easily. I was always so relieved to discover a chair or stool in any shop we went in. I would just sit on it and wait whilst Simon browsed. In the evening we visited new parents André and Claire, (they had a sofa, so that was no problem!).

The next day Jerry's wife Jenny very kindly took me to our local garden centre where we had lunch in their newly-refurbished restaurant. I needed a break after browsing around the many departments and eventually buying some items of clothing to cheer me up – I had to do this now before my money ran out! I also needed a rest because I couldn't walk very far for very long. It felt good to know that I was always with someone.

That week, Nick was involved with a project on behalf of the local Youth Club, whereby he did some work at a local park for the council – re-building steps, gardening, planting trees, tidying up, etc. So good and conscientious was he that the foreman suggested he should consider working for the council full time when he left school! As it happened, he worked for a large garden centre instead – close enough! He was even photographed at the Town Hall, with fellow student helpers, receiving a certificate of commendation from the Town Mayor in honour of his achievements, which was published in several local newspapers. Oh, some good news at last!

6/8/08: Attended Force for my massage but the massage therapist had me booked down for reflexology when I actually just wanted a normal head/back massage. I was particularly averse to having anyone touching my feet at this time because the chemo had been giving me gip there (as well as everywhere else!): they were getting red and sore around the toes – a bit like Toby's bad paw! Plus, I found it hard to believe that wouldn't tickle me! I was therefore given to another therapist for a "normal" massage (lavender oils on my back, etc.) Strangely, the therapist commented on what a lovely surname I had! I'd never had anyone say that before. It's usually repeated incorrectly as Gusgott, Guscutt; and once someone even rang up to ask for Mrs Gaspot! (I should have married a "Smith"!)

As I'm typing this, the number 7 on my keyboard has become loose – oh! Now it's come off completely! I hope I don't need to type that number now, or the ampus "and" above it! Oh dear...I've just realised: my next entry is for the *seventh* of August! Just my luck! Here goes:

7/8/08 (that's a bit of luck – Nick's fixed it for me!): Was due to attend the Oncology clinic at the hospital in the afternoon. However, had to ring in to say I was too ill to go, due to having a very bad headache (possibly migraine), a runny nose and was being sick.

The next day I awoke with a bad toothache (methinks I need a complete new body). However, I managed to attend hospital for my usual chemotherapy session. It transpired that my blood count was low – not enough white blood cells apparently. I was seen by the Oncologist's nice Registrar who explained that I was probably suffering from what is commonly known in the medical profession as an "anxiety attack" or "anticipatory sickness". Oh great! Now I was psychologically affected by physical events – I was going mental! It was therefore arranged for me to turn up again for chemo the following Monday. Whilst there, he also examined my mouth and teeth and I discovered it would probably complicate matters if I had to also attend a dentist to sort out my toothache – I'd have to explain about my chemo treatment, etc. which would affect any treatment, so I thought I'd just put up with it and hope it would go away – it certainly paled to insignificance compared with the excessive vomiting I was doing!

In the evening we gave our young friends' baby some presents. Later I suffered more from my very painful toothache.

As if that wasn't enough, whilst we were watching "Die Hard" on the TV, my car alarm went off! When we investigated it, the alarm didn't work at all! But then the next day it did! Huh? Was somebody just out to get me?

9/8/08: My tooth was still hurting.

That weekend Nick participated in a local Model Railways Exhibition in aid of an Air Ambulance Trust. One of his remote control tanks was displayed travelling around the model town in someone's back garden, as well as his steam engine and remote control car. There was a raffle, hosted by Dave, the Town Crier (who is also the Treasurer of our drama group) and we chatted with Chris, the newly-appointed Town Mayor, over coffee during a break in the proceedings. The event raised £1000! (the exhibition, not our chatting to the Mayor!)

Later, Zoe popped in to see how I was doing, which I thought was nice.

11/8/08: Was Simon's mum's 80th birthday. Unfortunately, it was also the day of my postponed chemo. I was moved around this time from room to room, chair to chair. Due to my constant vomiting, the side of my stomach was fitted with an anti-sickness syringe driver. It was a syringe fitted inside a half see-through box, powered by a C5 battery and attached via a very long tube (I looked even more like a robot now with all these tubes protruding from my body!). Every few seconds a whirring noise eminated from it as the syringe pumped the medication into my body. It was basically the "Zombie" drug (otherwise known as Nozinan) in liquid form. A female patient was in a bed opposite me (as opposed to large chairs, like the rest of us) and she was very unwell with stomach problems, awaiting a scan and she said she couldn't eat much. I told her that I had just discovered that, contrary to how I had interpreted eating instructions pre-chemo, I actually <u>was</u> allowed to eat cheese (eg cheddar) during chemo, just not the soft cheese like blue/stilton! As it happens, I don't really like cheese much anyway, so I didn't miss out much!

The auxilliary nurse was a welcome sight in the ward at midday, as usual, with a trolley full of free sandwiches. Unfortunately, I couldn't really have any as they prompted vomiting, especially so soon after the chemical injections. However, I managed to have lunch in one of the hospital restaurants at 3 o'clock, then left at 3.30. I found myself living on fruit (when my mouth wasn't sore – juice from an orange <u>stung</u> like crazy!), cup-a-soup and crisps (again, when my mouth was ulcer-free).

A district nurse visited daily to refill the "driver". On Thursday she had to remove the actual driver as there was a red mark around the insertion point. She said I would probably feel a "pea-like" lump there for approximately a week. She therefore inserted a new driver on the other side of my tummy. She also had to flush the Hickman line. I could feel the coldness of the liquid as it rushed via the tube into my skin - oh joy!

She asked how my lips were now; were they still sore? To which I replied that they weren't – that would happen the next week! She said I made her laugh. Well, that was short-lived because, when she had finished she disappeared into the kitchen to wash her hands. I suddenly heard a loud splashing noise coming from in there. Apparently, she had struggled with our peculiar taps to the point that she had turned them the wrong way, facilitating a large, fast flow of tap water to exit from them, which reverberated around the sink, hitting her in the chest! Fortunately, she took it in good humour.

The next day Nick was off helping André with some work on his new house in a nearby village, so I was left on my own all day, barring my usual visit by the district nurse. The red area from where the first driver had been removed was sore and now hurt a lot, especially if I bent over, even a little. I had to chase up the nurse's visit because she hadn't appeared by her usual time. I rang the county On Call Doctors who immediately passed the message on. She turned up very soon thereafter – apparently, she hadn't received the message to visit me to remove the driver. Simon let her in because I had decided to get dressed as the time was getting on. Then I returned downstairs and heard her in the kitchen washing her hands. Unfortunately, she got splashed again by our tap!

16/8/08: The District Nurse came at 11 am to remove my driver. She told me that, yesterday, she had read how the chat show host, Trisha Goddard, who had contracted cancer the same time as myself, still goes to the gym to take her mind off the illness. However, she continued, she obviously has a different type of chemo, so the nurse hoped that not all will follow suit! (I think she may particularly have had someone like me in mind!) After showering every morning I feel exhausted and have to lie down for half an hour – everything wears me out, so I've no chance at a gym!

The following week Nick fell ill – it started with a headache and then he was sick (coming out in sympathy with me?). He was poorly for about three days. Because of this I had to go to his school to pick up his GCSE results (and the less said about them, the better). I went after the District Nurse flushed my Hickman line again.

22/8/08: Our farmer friends popped in to pay for tickets to see "Flashdance the Musical" in Torquay in November (a trip arranged via my drama group). I was keeping my fingers crossed to be able to see it myself, as it was in the evening and a fair distance away, and I knew how tired I got as the evening drew close.

24/8/08: Their village held a "Duck Race/Cream Teas" event, which we promptly missed due to Simon wanting to watch the end of "The Sweeney" on TV! However, we managed to attend eventually, meeting up with a lot of friends who asked how I was. One of them, Jan (nice name!) a local singer, said she had heard that our drama group play went well and also informed me that there were, in fact, several people in the village who were Hospiscare drivers – talk about a small world!

Simon and I eventually went on to have tea and cake with Alan and Christine at their farm.

26/8/08: Had a visit from a lady from Hospiscare (the one with the same name as my wig!). During her visit, she informed me that the Oncology department of the hospital I attend won an award a couple of years ago for being the second best Oncology Department in the UK, beaten only by Edinburgh! That cheered me up somewhat! (winning an award, not being beaten by Edinburgh!)

I had a bad migraine the next day, which was unfortunate, as I also had to deal with the Building Control Inspector who came for a final inspection of our garage conversation into Nick's "den". He came at 2 o'clock then, after he went, I was sick three times that afternoon (at least I waited till he had gone!).

28/8/08: I was due to have my usual freebie massage at Force but I was too ill to go to that; however I felt well enough to attend the Oncology Clinic, when I also underwent my usual pre-chemo blood test. Unfortunately, I had to go through that twice as the nurse inadvertently placed the syringe containing my blood into a "sharps" bucket for disposal! I facetiously asked if she had been there when the award was won! She took it in good humour and asked if I wanted to shoot her now or tomorrow, to which I replied I was too tired!

The next day I drove Nick to the dentist for his six-monthly check-up, followed by a light lunch at a nearby pub/restaurant where one of Christine's two daughters works.

On the following Sunday Simon drove me to the coast again, which was nice.

1/9/08: 9.15 – 11.45: Had another chemo session after another blood test, due to a low blood count the previous Friday. I learned later that day that, apparently, there are 750,000 white blood cells to one drop of blood! Just thought I'd mention that! It certainly boggled my mind!

2/9/08: 9.00 am the District Nurse came to refill my syringe driver, and the next day she renewed it. She refilled it again on the 4th, then drew my blood and flushed my line the next day. Also that day I had a call from Gina, at Hospiscare, to ask if I needed a visit, which I thought was very kind, if unnecessary. I was sure there must have been other people who were in more of a need for her reassuring visits. Nevertheless, I told her about the sites on my stomach from the driver insertions – about how they were sore, lumpy, red blobs and she responded by calling me "Mrs Blobby"! Sympathetic or what?!

Do you know, it rained virtually every day since July and it was now September! Not that I really missed the non-existent summer – especially as I had been told to keep out of the sun or wear good sunblock if I ventured out (that was obviously assuming we would have sunny days!) I think there might have been at least one sunny day!

3/9/08: District Nurse came to renew syringe driver etc.

She did it the next day too.

She took a blood sample and flushed my line the next day.

7/9/08: Caroline, the Hospiscare-recommended home massage therapist rang me to arrange a free home massage for myself and Simon. This was great! I couldn't believe the pampering myself and my carer were getting! Just because I had cancer! I know that last sentence sounds strange but really, I just am constantly amazed at the support on offer for sufferers like myself and am extremely grateful.

8/9/08: I was lucky enough to be taken to hospital by Hospiscare Voluntary Transport (I tried to donate a small sum each time if I could afford it). My chemo appointment was actually 9.15 but I wasn't seen until 11 am. I didn't feel like reading a magazine so I just stared at the gigantic fish tank or gazed in wonderment at the huge, incomplete jigsaw laid out on one of the coffee tables. Radio 2 was playing on the radio on a window sill. One of the nurses went over the moon when she discovered one of the fish in the tank had had babies! Gradually, a small crowd of hospital staff gathered round the tank to see the sight!

I finally got called for treatment around 10.45 – just when a good song finally came on the radio! The male nurse asked if I wanted to stay then but I jumped up and followed him to the large, crowded, treatment room.

I vomited just before he commenced my treatment and he kindly went and got me a couple of Murray mints from the sweet tin to get rid of the taste!

I'm now having trouble with my wireless computer mouse as I type this. The red light keeps flashing. I accidentally knocked it on the floor just now and when I picked it up, the light had stopped flashing and now it's working fine! Technology! Huh! Back to my chemo visit:

The woman in the bed opposite to me chatted with me about my chemo whilst I was waiting to be seen. We both thought the room was very cold – in fact, all the patients did, to such a degree that we all needed coats and blankets! It was something to do with the heating being off at the weekend and taking a while to come back on again. I kept sneezing. I didn't know if it was to do with the chemo or the cold! However, the temperature in the toilet was even worse. As I came out and walked briskly back to my seat, rubbing my hands, I called out to everyone: "You all think this is cold – you should try the toilet!"

The nurse was inserting the syringe driver into my tummy which I wasn't too happy about for a different reason to usual: I was seated right next to a young man and his dad, who was sitting on a bed, both of whom had a clear view of the proceedings! I also vomited shortly afterwards (even after trying on anti-sickness wrist bands Christine had supplied!). I apologised to the two patients who told me not to worry. As they were leaving, shortly after, they informed me that the dad had a 10cm large tumour in his stomach which chemo wouldn't be able to help as it was much too large. I sympathised with them and wished them luck as they left.

Once my treatment had finished I wandered back to the waiting room where Trevor, my Hospiscare lift was waiting. A tall, mature man in a suit, reading a newspaper. He belongs to our county's Conservation

Trust, having previously been a member of the Rotary (I used to belong to the 18-30 Rotaract Group!) and is also a musician (organ). We made our way through the two corridors leading to one of the car parks and, as we entered the car, observed a young, distraught woman outside the Oncology department, being hugged closely by a man. She was in tears. I couldn't help but feel sorry for her. We drove off on our seventeen mile journey back home.

9/9/08: District Nurse attended me 9.30.

10/9/08: District Nurse attended me 9.30.

Simon surprised me that day with a dozen red roses! I was thrilled! (He rarely does this!)

11/9/08: District Nurse flushed my line.

12/9/08: I have lots of mouth ulcers now. The Difflam Oral Rinse given to me by the hospital takes ages to have any effect.

The directors of a local tank company invited Nick to go along to their tank exhibition, following the recent charity event he participated in. Nick was happy to attend.

That weekend Simon's older brother Chris and his partner Susan visited for lunch, on their way (to or from – I can't remember which) visiting her grandfather. Unfortunately, she has a detached retina in one of her eyes and she related to me the time a nurse informed her that, because of this, she could not go on a roller coaster, parachute jump or, wait for it, do boxing! Oh drat! During their visit, the conversation turned, at one point, to household chores such as ironing. We were told that she does ironing with the TV on, or with the radio on, or sometimes with nothing on!!

15/9/08: Had 38 "Get Well" cards now!

Had to take Nick to the dentist for a filling at 11.30.

Simon was in a playful mood today. He probably won't thank me for revealing the following but, what the hell! He called out to me from our newly-transformed guest room "Come and see this!" I walked in and couldn't see him anyway – and it's only a small room with a bed, chest of drawers and wardrobes in it. So I replied, in no particular direction, "You're not going to jump out suddenly from somewhere and say 'Boo!' are you?". Then I approached the airing cupboard next to the bed, opened the door (about three feet off the floor) and there he was, squatting at the bottom. He said "Boo!" in a childish manner. I sighed and walked away, trying not to smile, and wondering if he managed to extricate himself from the small space without hurting himself! He's as bad as Nick sometimes who, lately, has taken to backchatting in a cheeky way. For instance, every time he goes out of the house and I call to him "OK – take care", he replies: "Take care is my middle name...... Aaaaghhh!" and pretends to fall! Kids!

17/9/08: Gill, another of my drama group friends came round for lunch. I cooked lasagne for us. She gave me a lovely bunch of lilies which I displayed proudly on the table. At 2 pm Zoe called in with homemade cake and bread! I was getting spoilt that day!

The next day Irene rang for a chat and to see how I was getting on, so I told her.

My hair was finally starting to show proper signs of growing back (approximately one and a half millimetres so far! – Well, that's better than being completely bald!)

The following day the District Nurse came to flush my line.

21/9/08: Simon drove me to Dawlish, where we sat and ate fish and chips by the river that led to the sea. It was, surprisingly, a lovely sunny day. I even won three keyrings at the local amusements! Don't know what to do with them though.....they're slightly childish (a red, rubbery alien was one of them!)

22/9/08: Our oven stopped working. Simon needed a new cambelt for his Fiesta car and then he told me he was going to have to work Saturday, meaning I would have no help in preparing everything like meals etc. for our visitors who were due then. (We'd invited Alan and Christine, then Simon's parents wanted to come down the same weekend – we couldn't say no.) We had to hurriedly try to purchase and instal a new oven!

That evening, I tried to take my mind off these problems by being picked up by Gill to go to my drama group's committee meeting close by. I was pleased to hear the Treasurer's report, stating that we were in the black by nearly £1,000 – and after only two productions so far!

25/9/08:   1.50:   Had usual appointment to attend Oncology clinic before the next chemo session. Waited a long time to be seen, my back was facing the large TV screen but it was a programme I wouldn't have watched anyway.

The next day the District Nurse came to take the usual blood sample and flush the line. I just about remembered to give her the blood sheet prepared the previous day at the clinic. She also asked me to acquire certain medical items they were short of from the hospital on my next visit: blood test forms, pink cleaning skin stuff, Hepsal for line flushing and water for injection. Apart from that, things were getting slightly repetitive by now, albeit there's not much wrong with routine I suppose – especially when compared to horrible surprises, as happened later in the year! (q.v. later chapters)

CHAPTER SEVENTEEN

Happy Birthday To Me!

Simon's parents came to stay the weekend of twenty-seventh September (my number seven has completely given up the ghost now...). Alan and Christine came round to join us all for dinner Saturday evening, even bringing their own home-made clotted cream (well, they were *dairy* farmers!). Mum presented me with a home-made birthday cake made by our mutual friends Brenda and Alan (my birthday was due in several days – 4th October).

On the Sunday we took his parents for a carvery meal at a nearby Pub/ Restaurant.

29/9/08: Simon drove me to hospital for chemo again for my 9.15 appointment. I took my syringe driver with me to return to them, as it was agreed to now try the treatment without it. Whilst waiting for treatment, I became aware of another patient's problem with her nails (another side effect of chemotherapy, I understood), as well as a "burning" chest. Well, at least I didn't have *those* side-effects.

My hair was finally starting to grow. I was now no longer a "shiny slaphead" but a "stubbly skinhead"! However, if viewed in a bright light, it appeared to be returning in a grey colour. So I tried to look at it in darker lighting, where it appeared a darker colour!

Back home, Alix, the secretary at the Police Force, rang me to see how I was doing. So I told her. She remarked that she thought I was a "fighter" (referring to the cancer, of course!) Unfortunately, she was ringing from her bed as she had recently over-exercised at the gym, pulling a tendon on her leg. She told me that her boyfriend had wrapped a bandage over a packet of frozen peas on her leg – then burst it! He then left her to go running! Looked like I wasn't the only one with problems!

4/10/08:   My 50th birthday. I had hoped, last year, to have spent it in California but alas, this was not to be! However, I still had a good one – Simon bought me a dozen, large red roses and a bunch of gorgeous lilies, together with a long black coat and black leather handbag, and Nick surprised me by buying me pseudo-diamond drop-earrings! Alan and Christine dropped in with a birthday present and chocolate and a bunch of carnations, then Simon suddenly vanished only to re-appear soon after carrying a chocolate birthday cake which, despite having decorated it himself with my name only seconds earlier, looked quite neat!

They all sang "Happy Birthday" before each having a piece! I also had several phone calls from friends and relatives, including my aunt June in America! My uncle Bill told me I was a fighter (I'm beginning to get a complex about that!) and alert, and that it was all to do with the mind as well.

At 12.30 the plumber arrived (nothing to do with my birthday) to check the central heating thermostat. He didn't stay long.

To top it all, Simon had apparently arranged for us to have a lavish meal at 8 pm at the posh hotel/restaurant in the countryside where we had all celebrated Christine's birthday earlier in the year. I had a lovely time, even though I was hoping, all the while, that my wig would stay straight! As usual, I had no desire for alcohol but didn't miss it.

CHAPTER EIGHTEEN

Living Life in the Slow Lane

6/10/08: I vomited at chemo again. Vincent, the male nurse administering the treatment, thought he had discovered what triggered it – he said it was, ironically, probably due to me having the "anti-sickness" drug which is given prior to the chemo!

Nurse Alison overheard me discussing my birthday treat at the posh Restaurant and – talk about a small world – apparently she had been a guest at the evening wedding reception being held in the adjacent hall and marquee!

On the way home after chemo, as we were driving up the fast dual-carriageway, Trevor, my Hospiscare driver, pointed to something in the distance saying "Isn't that pretty?" I could only see the surrounding fields and motorway signs.

"What?" I asked, "The motorway sign?"

He laughed and explained he was referring to the autumn colours of leaves on a big tree we passed. I guess I missed that; probably due to my post-chemo drowsiness.

7/10/08: I heard our drama group had been given £100 grant from the local council! Hooray!

That weekend, I went with Simon and Nick to have their photos taken professionally. I just wanted something nice to look at when I was alone at home and suffering (boo hoo!) – also, I was fast running out of my savings, spending it on bills, and I wanted something to show for it once it had all been used up. After a lot of nice shots of the two of them, the photographer suggested I join them in a group shot, but I wasn't keen (a) because I was wearing a wig and my SOS talisman necklace, which would only serve to remind me that I had cancer at the time and (b) I had absolutely no make-up on, and whenever I have no make-up on, I look ill even when I'm well, so let alone now – when I *am* ill – if you see what I mean.....Anyway, I reluctantly obliged and the framed photos now take pride of place in our lounge, although I try to steer any viewings away from the ones with me in them!

In the afternoon, Simon drove me to a couple of local resorts. Whilst at one of them, we noticed crowds of people gathering nearing the sloping shingle beach and wondered what was going on as there was nothing obvious. It wasn't long before we heard the sound of an aeroplane approaching, fairly low, and it turned out to be a genuine Spitfire, flying overhead to commemorate (we later discovered) a chap who recently died, who was a "pillar of the community", or some such thing, due mainly to his organising an annual festival or something.

In the next village stop we encountered the statue of Sir Walter Raleigh.

Then we went home. The weather wasn't particularly nice.

Sunday we popped into our local inn for a quick drink – well, I had a coke because, as you must know by now, I wasn't allowed alcohol with chemo. My old school friend, Heather, had rung earlier in the day to ask if she and her husband Gary could call in on their way back from Cornwall on the 25th.

When I mentioned about the alcohol she replied: "Blimey! The one time you actually need a drink and you're not allowed it!"

When I rang her back some time later, she wasn't available, only Gary, and I told him it would be OK to see us after their trip as we would be home. We chatted for a while and he said he'd get her to ring me back.

Unfortunately, when she did, she informed me that their Cornish trip was meant to be a birthday surprise for Gary and I'd let the cat out of the bag! However, she had managed to quell his suspicions but I somehow don't think I'll be allowed to forget it!

At this time, I kept having dreams about having long, dark hair (well, pretty much what I had before this all began) and was then disappointed, on waking up, to see that I was still a "skinhead" (better than a "slaphead", I suppose!) Nick also referred to my new look as akin to a hedgehog! Thanks Nick!

13/10/08: I was cheered up by attending the local town council offices where a meeting was being held in the evening, presided over by the Town Mayor. The local press was there too, all in aid of the presentation of certificates to the five Youth Club members who had given up their free time to work voluntarily at the local park, including Nick of course. The councillor who was primarily involved made a little speech about each of them before the Mayor handed over their certificates and they posed for photos. I was particularly proud to hear his comments about Nick, that he worked hard no matter what the weather. I naturally had to take some photos myself!

Whilst I was waiting with Simon before the proceedings, I was approached by Lyn, the town clerk and Vernon, the ex-Mayor of the previous year, who both asked how I was doing, which was nice. I knew them in my capacity as founder of the local drama group. In fact, Vernon had kindly attended the inaugural meeting of the group the previous year which had, no doubt, helped to boost numbers!

CHAPTER NINETEEN

Go With the Flow...

Simon had been thinking, for some time, of having his own business, i.e. a shop or even a market stall. We both, therefore, started looking into renting a shop in the high street but, after further investigation, decided against it due to the expensive rates. Still, it made a change from worrying about cancer.

I noticed, anyway, that – of late – I was beginning to feel much better – probably due to the less potent treatment I was receiving. I didn't vomit half as much and not for half as long! Although I still kept my eyes peeled for seats to sit on during any shopping sprees for when I felt tired. Despite that, I was actually beginning to feel a sense of normality about my life and hoped it would last; it was such a welcome relief.

15/10/08: We eagerly flicked through the pages of our local newspapers and found a colour photo of Nick and his group there, together with a write up!

16/10/08: Bashed into Terry, the manager of the local market, whilst we were out shopping and made enquiries about having a market stall but, like all our other plans and ambitions, this soon died a death a few weeks later. The thought of standing around a stall in the cold wind and rain didn't do much to encourage the idea. Oh well....I was getting used to this.

I had a phone call that day from Hospiscare, to check up on me as usual. They said they would ring again in a couple of weeks.

In the last few weeks, I noticed Nick and Simon kept stroking my head whilst I was sitting on the sofa, because my new hair was so soft, like a baby's! It continued for some time!

17/10/08: It was Brenda's birthday.

The District Nurse visited in the morning (I can't remember why, but they usually had some reason).

Saturday 19th I felt up to having lunch with Simon at the local wine bar where Tracey, one of the members of our drama group worked.

That day, whilst queuing a long time at the checkout in Boots, Simon put his arm around me then kissed me, totally unexpectedly! I must have looked bored (before he kissed me, not after!) He obviously didn't give two hoots about everyone else in the queue watching us! He did something similar outside a posh department store where we used to live: I had told him I would visit another shop while he entered the department shop then, in the very busy pedestrianised high street, he suddenly grabbed me, swung me round and pulled me towards him, giving me a big smacker on the lips whilst holding me tight! I thought that sort of thing only happened in the movies! He's a man of few words but by golly, do his actions make up for it!! I suppose secretly I'm quite pleased! It's as if we've only just met but we celebrated our 18th wedding anniversary the following March.

20/10/08: Nick received 46 mobile phone messages, most of which he couldn't be bothered to answer. He said most of them, but not all, were from ten girls who liked him! Honestly, it's like living with a pop star sometimes.

Nick was in a playful mood that Sunday evening: I was struggling to put clothes away in the airing cupboard in the spare room when he called to me from our bedroom "Quick! Go in your bedroom! There's been an accident!" I couldn't be bothered to go. I knew what he was like for pranks and practical jokes – pretty much like his father! So he continued: "Hurry up or he'll die!" Now bear in mind Nick was all of 16 years old when this happened....So I ambled across the landing into our bedroom and what did I see? On our bed was a soft, cuddly teddy bear (OK, I own up – he usually takes pride of place on our pillows and we call him Fred Bear!) whose head had been squashed underneath my laptop, on top of which was a hand written note saying "HELP!" Honest!

21 and 22/10/08: Simon was lucky enough to be granted an interview at a local Marks and Spencer Simply Food store at 10 am. That evening he was offered the job of Customer Services Assistant. I was so pleased for him. He had been wanting to get out of the building industry for some time due mostly to health reasons (he's getting old you know!). That evening he visited the GP surgery to check out problems he was having with his arm. Turned out it was "tennis elbow" and an appointment was made for him to visit a physiotherapist some time later. So now we were both ill! Still, we had a meal at the local inn to both celebrate his new job and cheer us up regarding our health – only one course though, and it was one of the last times we could go as we were both getting poorer! I was obviously unemployed due to my cancer treatment and Simon would now be on a much lower wage.

23/10/08: I was wearing a new, long, grey woollen cardigan I hadn't worn before. It had a very large collar. And I mean *very* large! It hugged my neck and the tips of it almost reached my stomach! Simon said it made me look like Darth Vader from Star Wars!

1.50: I had an appointment at the Oncology Clinic again. I actually decided to leave home when I felt like it because I was always kept waiting two to three hours, even if I arrived early. I was seen by a doctor other than the Oncologist – whom I had only seen once. (Must have been something I said!) I was informed of the following:

Apparently, according to my previous blood samples, my liver appeared to be doing badly during the first sessions involving the Epirubiscin, which was the very strong chemical. It was suggested I had an ultrasound but, for now, being that I was on milder chemotherapy (CMF), my liver was good and my kidney and blood were very good. Also my white blood cells. I mentioned my red, blotchy feet but was informed this was most probably a rash due to the chemo. The doctor didn't realise I was due to have a mastectomy later down the line and advised that it would need to be (at least) twelve months before I could have reconstructive surgery and it was a very big operation. She informed me that they would only do reconstructive surgery if I was not overweight and added that the extra weight I said I had put on in the last few months was only due to the chemo. I told her I was relieved because I thought it was due to all the extra food I had been eating – I was always hungry lately, possibly due to excessive vomiting leaving me empty all the time!

She mentioned that the cancer itself was always very low and small, however chemo was needed due to the lymph glands problem, which was more severe. She concluded by telling me they would continue to need to see me for the next five years. Again I was relieved. This time because, on one of my chemo sessions, I "accidentally" read my medical notes when the nurse had to go somewhere and I, naturally, didn't understand much of the terminology. I got as far as a sheet which started talking about the type of cancer I had (some long words) and mentioned the words "five years". This struck terror in my heart because I assumed it was referring to how long I had left to live! I had to stop reading at that point because the nurse came back. I told the doctor this and she smiled reassuringly: "No, no....that is how long we need to keep seeing you for before you can get the "all clear". However, you will still need to have regular mammograms and check yourself as before..."

24/10/08: The plumber came to have a look at our boiler which was going wrong.

Shortly afterwards the District Nurse visited to do the flushing and take a blood sample. That is, she was meant to. She was accompanied by an NHS nurse who, apparently, hadn't had much experience at phlebotomy. Unfortunately, neither had the District Nurse, so they couldn't get a blood sample. Still, whilst flushing my line, we discussed my whole attitude to my condition. They told me that having a positive attitude, such as I had apparently, could help cure cancer by up to 50%! Something to do with the endorphines in your system that are released when one has such an attitude/laughed a lot. Well I certainly laughed a lot – though not whilst vomiting. Anyway, that cheered me up! They backed it up by relating a recent case they had been dealing with concerning a young woman who had cancer from her knees to her toes. Unfortunately, she had been living with a particularly violent partner. However, once he left her, she immediately became happier and her health consequently improved. The nurse said the release of endorphines was definitely a contributory factor!

Later that day I was interviewed over the phone by Anita of the local City newspaper, regarding Hospiscare. The paper was doing a series of articles over a month, specifically about cancer (called "Cancer Aware Month") and, apparently, Angela of Hospiscare had suggested myself to speak to her because the paper wanted someone "chatty". Can't think why they chose me!! Anyway, I was grateful for the opportunity to mention my thanks for all the support I had been given by various organisations, including, of course, Hospiscare, Force Cancer Support, Macmillans Nurses, GP, District Nurses, the Breast Care Nurses and other staff at the hospital plus family and friends (hope I haven't forgotten anyone!). I had no idea there was so much support out there for sufferers like myself and I wanted people to know that Hospiscare is not just associated with terminally-ill patients (as I had hitherto thought) but, in fact, have a lot to offer people like myself, including (not least) constant support both in person and on the phone – people to talk to, help with transport to and from hospital, even home massage therapy treatments! Then I mentioned this book I'm writing and she said to let them know when it's finished (chance would be a fine thing!) and she would help advertise it in their paper for me!

25/10/08:   Heather and Gary popped in, as planned, on their way back from Cornwall for lunch (we're quite strategically placed between the south west and their home in Essex!) The subject of my faux pas was naturally discussed and laughed about. Fortunately, Gary made me feel a little better about it by saying that, because I had let the cat out of the bag early, he was able to spend the time beforehand actually looking forward to it rather than having it suddenly sprung on him! (Thanks Gary!)

Our town's annual carnival took place that evening but they had a long journey ahead of them so they didn't attend. Neither did we – it was too much of a hectic event for me to consider attending in my condition.

Noon, the next day, Simon and I were treated to our Hospiscare massages by Caroline.

27/10/08: One of my last chemo sessions at 10.45. Simon was able to attend with me this time. I only vomited once in the hospital – unfortunately, it was pretty bad – I was holding the grey, cardboard sick tray underneath my mouth to catch the fluid. (I hope you're not eating as you're reading this). I caught the fluid alright, but I couldn't catch my breath; I was choking on my own vomit, gasping in between exuding regurgitated lumps of bread and liquid. It seemed to go on forever. For a few seconds my mind was racing with thoughts of unwanted death, in between trying to breathe. I didn't want to die in hospital in this embarrassing way – I didn't want to die at all. Simon, who had been sitting beside me, immediately jumped up and came round to me. The male nurse, who had been sitting in front of me with the tray of syringes on his lap, stood before me and calmly told me to try to breathe slowly. It was all I could do to breathe at all. Finally, the feeling subsided. There was no more vomit and I was able to breathe properly again. I used to feel a lot better and relieved after "vomit sessions" but this time I just felt exhausted.

Moments later, another nurse appeared and told my nurse that the family opposite, particularly the young woman, asked to be moved into the adjacent treatment room - I gathered because they couldn't stand sitting opposite someone (albeit about five yards away!) who was being sick. I don't blame them really. Although it didn't make me feel very good to be scaring people away!

I took some sick trays with me for the journey back home. I felt reasonable for most of the journey but when we were about two minutes from our house in Simon's car, I struggled to hold back an overwhelming desire to be sick again. I grabbed hold of a sick tray as we approached a mini-roundabout. That was it. I couldn't contain it any more – a whole load of vomit poured from my mouth as Simon negotiated the roundabout. As he continued up the hill past it, I found myself struggling to breathe again. All he could say was "Don't spill it in the car!" I don't think he realised I couldn't breathe. He pulled the car over into a slight layby before the brow of the hill, telling me to tip the contents out near the grassy knoll. My breathing gradually improved as I did as instructed and we continued on our way. I was exhausted again and couldn't wait to get in and just lie down. Fortunately, I only experienced a few more bouts that day, not necessitating the need to stay in bed for a week, like I used to a few months previously.

28/10/08:   Simon started his new job.

29/10/08:   The newspaper photographer came round to take my photograph for the Hospiscare article. As it was (unusually) a sunny day, he opted to take it in our long, busy back garden. I wore my wig, of course, and he asked me to pose by the side of our white-walled garage, the side of which was adjacent to, and formed part of, our garden. It was separated by a path, with plants, bushes, a patio area and a small pond on the other side, which eventually led to more plants, trees, bushes, garden ornaments, statues (all left behind by the previous owners). Being autumn, it didn't look its best, but there was still a bit of colour around on some of the plants. Unfortunately, he got me facing the sun, so my photo makes me look like a Chinese woman squinting in order to see! I was hardly wearing any make up and my wig just made my face look chubby and puffy (as opposed to quite slim without the wig – being a skinhead has its advantages!) Still, I think I looked quite happy, considering!

It was developed quite quickly, as the whole article was in the next day's edition! It was a whole page and, embarrassingly, my colour photo was larger than I expected – I thought it would be the size of a passport photo but, instead, it was at least six times bigger! My chubby face was there for all to see – hopefully more notice would be taken of my words than my face!

The article itself was accurate barring when the journalist wrote that I had suffered the odd "blip" during chemo. What?! Is that what you call it? I supposed they didn't want to alarm anyone.

That evening I was sitting in the lounge watching TV when I overheard a brief conversation between Simon and Nick (who were by the fridge in the adjacent kitchen) which went something like:

Simon: What's this?

Nick: It's chocolate I bought for mum....Galaxy – but I ate most of it!

I didn't know whether to laugh or cry!

31/10/08: The District Nurse came for the usual flushing/bloods (an experienced one this time!)

3/11/08: My chemo session again. It had been arranged for a different Hospiscare driver to take me – Mary, the wife of Trevor. She was meant to pick me up at 9.30 am for a 10.15 appointment. At about 9.40 I looked out of my window and could see a car I didn't recognise parked in the street opposite. A lady got out and walked up the path of a nearby house. Moments later she appeared and drove away only to reappear on the other side of that road, parking outside one of the bungalows. She knocked on that door too before returning to the car. She didn't get back in. Instead, she produced a mobile phone and stood by the car, looking all around while she was talking on it. It wasn't hard to guess who she was, even though I had never seen her before! I went to my door, stood there and waved but she didn't see me standing alongside a hedgerow and large bushes. So I went back indoors to get my coat and handbag and went back outside. This time I walked down the few steps and stood on our driveway beside the hedgerow, waving again to attract her attention. She was looking the other way. Finally I caught her eye and she got back in the car, driving it up to our house, parking near the drive. She got out and asked if I was Jan Guscott, apologising profusely, obviously embarrassed by the whole incident, even though Trevor had given her directions to our house! I told her not to worry but it gave us something to talk about at the beginning of the half-hour journey.

With this new lot of chemicals I was on, although they weren't as potent, it did mean more frequent trips to hospital. I was also warned that the effect would be cumulative and because of that, at the very end of that treatment, I would feel even more tired than I was already.

At this time, there was a viral infection in eight of the wards, so visitors were advised to keep away from those specific wards. Various hospital entrances were either closed off or supervised where previously they hadn't been. They were obviously trying to contain the situation. Fortunately, my chemo ward was unaffected. I entered through two lots of double doors, approached the receptionist and announced myself as usual:

"Hi, 'Vomit Woman' here again!"

And so began my next lot of treatment and vomiting!

Whilst nurse Vincent was pumping me full of chemicals I commented on our hair similarities. I was wearing my full wig of course and he had a very short haircut:

"I've got nearly as much hair as you now!" I said, grinning. Well, at least I was no longer completely bald, even though he couldn't see it!

One of the other patient's husband kindly offered me a cup of tea but I politely declined, aware of what that might prompt in my body. I was already feeling nauseous. Didn't make any difference though – I still vomited eventually, as usual. I was attached to a saline drip, feeling like a baby with a bib! An hour or so later Mary drove a weary me back home.

7/11/08: The District Nurse came for her regular visit. Then Simon and I had lunch at the local tea rooms in town.

Later that day the interior of my mouth felt like metal. Eating an Indian curry was painful – every mouthful stung like crazy. Nick commented that, by the time my chemo had finished, I would be turning into "Robocop" because of the metal feeling!

I heard, the next day, of the sad news of the death of Chris, our Town Mayor. He passed away at his home following a heart operation. Jerry, our Vice-Chairman remarked that it was a "double blow" as he had been "all for us" as a group. I felt sorry for his widow, whom I had met at the recent Charity do, and sent her a Sympathy card on behalf of our group as well as signing the Book of Condolence at the Town Hall. Although I hadn't known him very long, I thought Chris had been a really nice man who will be greatly missed.

CHAPTER TWENTY

Light at the End of the Tunnel

Monday, 10/11/08: I had a meeting at our house with Jerry, mainly to discuss auditions for the next play, a "whodunnit" by Agatha Christie. I thought it was about time we took on something more challenging! I just hoped it would work out! At the time of writing I'm still keeping my fingers crossed!

The next day I took Nick for a driving lesson on private land at the farm. He was doing really well (all that quad experience I expect, plus the fact that he had a Puch Magnum moped when he was six, which he drove around our friend Nigel's farm). I took him again two days later. I popped into the Senior Citizens Centre to sort out my Council Tax forms (necessary to apply for benefit).

14/11/08: This was not only Prince Charles' birthday, but also my younger brother Stephen's birthday, as well as my aunt June's in America. My mother always told me I was just like her in many ways – in looks as well as ways – not necessarily flattering ones, either. For instance, I discovered I share her dislike of sewing, particularly small items such as buttons! However, I make up for it in other ways such as sharing her great sense of humour and joy of life, in spite of everything!

Got 42 "Get Well" cards now! However, the newest ones were usually from the same people asking for an update of my health.

The District Nurse visited again.

Dad and Steve visited me that weekend. Steve showed me the book he had been working on which he had yet to finish (I think we're having a bit of a race now, to see who will finish their book first!). It was actually my mother's biography, which I began many years previously, prior to my meeting Simon. Unfortunately, that meeting kind of changed my life and intentions. Therefore, Steve kindly took over the writing. We had lunch in our favourite tea rooms in town on Saturday, followed by a carvery dinner at a pub/restaurant in a nearby village. In the evening we played pool at our local inn. On the Sunday Steve visited Alan's farm to help with research for his book (you'll have to read his book if you want to have that explained!).

Dad and Steve left Monday morning to head for Wales. They planned to return here the following week before going home to Hertfordshire.

The next day I booked Hospiscare transport for 24th November and 1st December – my very last chemo session! Hooray! Couldn't believe I was nearly there! Simon said he couldn't wait for me to get rid of my "plumbing" as he called my Hickman line!

The following evening, Christine and her friends picked me up from home to meet the coach at 5.30 taking my drama group and friends to Torquay to see "Flashdance, the Musical" at the Princess Theatre.

Before the performance I was able to distribute to members of our group the DVDs of our last performance.

I was slightly apprehensive about whether or not I would be able to stay awake during the evening, due to the tiredness I always experienced at that time of night. But I needn't have worried. The musical was so good (and some of the cast so good-looking!) – not to mention lively and envigorating – that I had no trouble staying awake; especially as we were seated only three rows back and immediately in front of the largest speakers you've ever seen! They must have been ten foot high if they were an inch! Plus three feet wide!

The long journey home was fairly noisy due to everyone discussing what they had just seen. I asked Jerry if he could make the announcements concerning future meetings, as I felt too tired.

20/11/08: Simon was reduced to tickling me in order to get me out of bed in the mornings! Karen, the local church Curate called in for her copy of the DVD and stayed for a cup of tea. We inevitably discussed my condition.

Later that day I had a visit (at 1.50 pm) to the Oncology department at the hospital for a chat about future procedures now that the chemotherapy was almost at an end. I saw Dr Goodman who told me to expect to have a mastectomy within the first two weeks of the following January. He told me I should receive a letter of confirmation to that effect quite soon from Mr Ferguson, the surgeon. Then, approximately three weeks later, in February, I should have radiotherapy lasting three weeks (excluding weekends). I was a bit surprised by this as I had originally been led to believe it would only last two weeks, not three, but Dr Goodman confirmed most emphatically that it would be three weeks. Thereafter I would need to wait at least six months before any reconstructive surgery could take place. Well, at least that was better than two years, as I had originally been told. I kept getting conflicting information.

Before I left, I asked if he knew how my treatment was going; in other words, I wanted to know if I had been going through all my pain and discomfort for nothing. He replied that scans can't show half centimetre or smaller sized tumours. Therefore I just had to let the hospital know if I got any unusual pain (not, for example, temporary backache or similar) – as this could be recurring cancer cells.

21/11/08: Simon bought a couple of ferrets for Nick. Despite the fact that they were Gills (girls), Nick still named them Spongebob and Patrick!

I had lunch that day with Christine, Jan (the local, professional singer) and Joan. Christine drove us to a nice, quiet inn in a harbour town some miles along the coast. We had a pleasant lunch before returning home, in time for mine and Simon's home massage, via Caroline, courtesy of Hospiscare. She put on a CD which played soothing music and we both felt all the better after our sessions, which took place in the master bedroom. To have used the bed in the guest room would have been ill-advised, as Simon pointed out, due to the fact that the large, antique pine double bed was too low for Caroline to bend over to massage us. He said, if she had done so, then *she* would have needed a massage afterwards, probably for a bad back!

Steve and dad came back the next day to pick up Steve's book, which I had managed to read during their absence. I drove Simon the mile to work that day (he didn't start till 11.45 am – I couldn't have done it if he had started earlier!) and picked him up 8pm. Later I saw Christine at the farm where I also gave Nick another driving lesson.

6 pm the next day dad and Steve went home.

24/11/08:   I was pleasantly surprised to see my Hospiscare driver today was a lady I knew from the nearby local village, who used to be a nurse, named Ada. My appointment was at 10.15. We chatted en route about her life in the village, which was full of lovely thatched cottages. Unfortunately, her husband had left her many years previously, with a disabled son, but she was coping admirably and enjoying her life. Well, the village residents saw to that; it's one of the nicest places I've ever been, with some of the nicest people. Christine and Alan lived there! (They moved whilst this book was in the making....ironically only a few streets from our house!)

A miracle occurred that day at the hospital: I didn't vomit once! Not even when I returned home.

27/11/08:   In the evening, Don, the Treasurer of the local Writers' Circle, kindly gave me a lift to a meeting in town with some publishers at the local library. Unfortunately, due to my breathlessness, he had to keep waiting for me to catch up with him once we left the car, even though he's quite a few years older than me! He's obviously quite fit for his age but left me feeling like an old lady because I felt so tired, especially as it was now evening; my usual "feeling exhausted" time of the day.

It was quite embarrassing once inside. Some of the members gathered around me, stopping me from acquiring refreshment for myself, insisting on getting it for me and then insisting on returning my empty cup! Several asked how I was doing, so I told them. I felt like an invalid! I suppose, in a way, I was. Anyway, the meeting was interesting but when I returned home I was very tired.

28/11/08:   The District Nurse did my bloods and flushing in the morning.

29/11/08:   Feeling a little better, though still weak if I walked too far, Simon took me out for a meal after dropping Nick off to see (one of) his girlfriend(s)!

The next day Jerry took me to see an Agatha Christie production by a tiny, local church group, which was interesting, albeit full of prompting near the end (but who am I to criticise?)

1/12/08:   Could it be – was it finally here - my final chemo treatment?! I was elated! And the icing on the cake was that, once again, I didn't vomit! I couldn't believe it! Trevor drove me to the hospital where, as before, one of the patient's relatives kindly offered to get me a drink, but I didn't dare take a chance – I wanted to maintain my new "non-vomiting" record, albeit brief!

The young Matron was treating me this time. Her name badge read "Collette". She looked nothing like Hattie Jacques, with whom I usually associate matron-types. She was very young, I thought, for someone in that position, small, slim with short dark hair (gone are the days of white paper-like hats and check dresses, she was in uniform scrubs like the rest of the staff, just a different colour – dark blue). She closed the curtains around me. The nurses had discovered that there was less likelihood of me vomiting if I prepared for such an event by concealing myself from other patients to avoid embarrassing all concerned, fate being the contrary thing that it is.

Whilst injecting the liquid chemicals into my Hickman line, she complimented my response to the whole cancer treatment, saying I was doing "brilliantly", which cheered me up, whether it was true or not! She remarked that I should now be seeing the "light at the end of the tunnel".

My mind turned to thoughts of religion and I replied:

"Hopefully not the light!"

"No," she giggled, "Not that light!"

When she had finished I asked her when I would be able to have my line removed and she told me she would try to find out and ring me at home. Later, at home, she advised me that there were only a couple of nurses qualified to remove it and one of them would perform the minor op. on 22nd December (just before Christmas, I thought – good timing!)

2/11/08:   The Writers' Circle was holding their annual get-together meal, to which Simon and I were both invited, at a lovely hotel several miles away in the country. Unfortunately, I was much too ill to attend due to the previous day's chemo treatment. I offered our apologies.

The next day I was admiring a photo on our calendar of a seaside town called "Beer". I didn't notice Nick pouring himself a drink of cherryade at the time. Still staring at the photo I remarked, absently, "I didn't realise that that was Beer...", to which he replied, quick as a flash as usual, "It's not beer, it's cherryade!"

4/11/08:   I sent a "Thank You" card to all the staff at the Chemotherapy Ward.

Nick visited the Minor Injuries Unit today following a recommendation by one of our local GPs, due to suspected tonsillitis and glandular fever. (We weren't a very healthy family at this time, but worse was to come....)

CHAPTER TWENTY-ONE

The Vanishing Staff

Friday, 5th December: After the usual visit from the District Nurse, Simon took me shopping to a village five miles away. He used my silver Mondeo as it was more comfortable than his Fiesta and could hold more shopping. I was quite tired and, as usual, had to sit down in every shop. I felt like an old lady again!

After about an hour, at 1 pm, we decided to have some lunch at a nice little cafe there, called the Bay Tree Café. Well, that is, we tried to!

There were half a dozen tables inside, all fully occupied bar one. So we sat there and ordered our two course lunch. I had soup for starters – vegetable, I think. I can't remember what Simon had, or even if he had any starter. The soup was delicious. Then came the main course; eggs, beans and chips. I remember looking beyond Simon to the elderly couple on the table behind and at the large windows beside them, which seemed a little steamy. I commented on how hot I was beginning to feel, assuming it was either something "menopausal", to do with eating hot food, or just the effect from the nearby kitchen several feet behind me.

A few minutes later I began to feel a bit dizzy . Moments later I said I felt faint. The next thing I knew I found myself waking up with the side of my face on my plate of food, staring at a large pool of yellow vomit on the table. I could feel Simon standing behind me, trying to sit me up, his hand on my forehead to keep me from falling back onto the plate, but I kept saying I wanted to sleep. Someone, presumably the waitress I thought, removed the plate. I sensed a lot of people gathering around me. My arms felt very weak – I had no energy, I just felt extremely tired. I heard someone say "Shall we get an ambulance?".

I eventually said to Simon, in a slow, drunken-like drawl "We've got to pay for our meal..."

I saw a glass of water on the table that wasn't there before, near my large, full cup of tea. I was helped to a sip of tea.

I noticed a woman at the doorway who was apparently on the lookout for the ambulance that had been called.

Simon left me for a few minutes to pay for the meal but I still felt sick – I tried to call to him, not very audibly. He didn't hear. I vomited again. He came back, using paper towels to mop up the mess, putting them into a big, black plastic bag.

I was so weak. I kept lowering my head and Simon kept holding my forehead saying "Stay with me Janice". I told you one day he would be my 'rock'.

I saw the remains of vomit on my light blue, zippy jumper and black jeans. (I no longer own them.) I could feel Simon removing some of it from my face just as the paramedics arrived; a man and a woman. The woman got Simon to help raise my feet onto another chair. She asked what had happened and how long I was out for. It was no good asking me – I was curious myself! Simon replied "only a few seconds". She took my pulse and called to her colleague that my blood pressure was very low – 94. She pricked my finger to test my blood's glucose level, etc., then asked me to squeeze her hands as tightly as I could. I made a feeble attempt, but could barely manage it as my arms were so weak. I told her about my left arm and lymph glands removal so she couldn't take blood pressure and the like from that arm. She noticed my "SOS" talisman necklace and I mumbled about how all my information was in that.

Then she and Simon struggled to get the elastic of an oxygen mask over my head without removing my wig!

"This is like being on the TV programme "Casualty"" I remarked, my voice obviously muffled through the mask.

Her colleague, who was standing at a nearby table, making notes, replied: "Not really – if it was, the window would be smashed and there'd be broken glass everywhere!"

I kept expressing how embarrassed and sorry I was for causing all this commotion but the kind waitress and her husband (the cook) told me not to worry.

The male paramedic took our names and address details, etc. We explained that I had had my last chemo the previous Monday – I commented on how pleased I had been not to vomit at that time but that I was now making up for it! I don't know how audible my voice was through the oxygen mask!

I heard bits of conversation between the customers to the effect that they saw an ambulance go straight past the café, presumably confusing the building with that of a nearby pub with a similar name! But they did turn up eventually. Two middle-aged ambulancemen entered the café, asking the same questions as the paramedics. I watched them trying to move the now-empty tables to make space for a stretcher.

I was still very weak and almost slurring my words with fatigue.

Whilst waiting, the waitress and her husband addressed me. Again I expressed my embarrassment and apologies to them. I said I hoped I hadn't put people off their food – it was disconcerting to see the sudden absence of customers in the last few minutes. I didn't even see them leave. But they reiterated their understanding of the situation, even in so far as telling me that I was more than welcome to return to the café when I was better (and I did)! The waitress told me that all their customers were regulars anyway and that one of them, Hazel, had even rushed out to go to the local doctor's surgery for me!

I kept falling back into Simon's chest, feeling the warmth of his sweater against my head, inducing the ever-present desire to sleep. But he held my head up, telling me to stay awake.

I don't remember getting on the stretcher. I said, again, that I was sorry if I put anyone off their food but the staff reassured me again, telling me not to worry because they were all regulars.

Simon went back to my car in order to be ready to follow the ambulance.

I said I felt a little better now and somebody therefore removed the oxygen mask.

I remember being wheeled, on the stretcher, out of the café and onto the narrow pavement. It seemed congested. My eyes fell on a silver car queueing behind the ambulance ramp. It was the first in a long line of cars. Apparently I was holding up all the traffic, which couldn't get past the ambulance because of the narrow road.

The ambulancemen wheeled me on board the ambulance.

Once inside, I commented to the friendly, red-haired one (not that the other one wasn't friendly!):

"I'm holding everyone up – is it me causing this?"

Unfazed, he replied:

"Don't worry – it's not your fault – we do this all the time!".

He strapped me in to prevent me falling out – at least that's the reason he gave!

"We often have to collect patients out of restaurants," he reassured me, "What we do is call out to the customers 'Don't eat the chicken!'"

He took my blood pressure. I told him the paramedic had already done that and he said they have to continually monitor it. Apparently it was a little better now – 108 instead of 94.

The ambulance doors were still wide open as the ramp was brought back inside. I caught a glimpse of the nice, female paramedic, who was frantically waving goodbye to me from the pavement, wishing me well. I just about managed to give her a limp goodbye wave with my weak arm.

I noticed the interior of the amulance seemed very modern – apparently it was only a couple of years old. The ambulanceman had a pen and forms in his hand and asked me what had happened, confirming my details. He kept making me laugh with a lot of silly comments, too numerous to mention here. (OK, I've forgotten them because I wasn't really 'with it' at the time!)

He said I sounded drunk because I was slurring my words. But I was just so tired. I replied that I wouldn't have minded but I sounded drunk without the benefit of alcohol beforehand! I added that I hadn't been allowed to consume alcohol during my chemotherapy treatment.

During the journey I slurred words to the effect that I thought all people in the health service should be paid a lot of money (I was so grateful for being looked after).

"But we don't", came the despondent reply.

It was a slightly bumpy ride. Due to my horizontal position, all I could see through the windows were tree tops.

We eventually arrived at the hospital (some 12 miles away) at approximately 1.30 pm. They parked outside the "Accident & Emergency" entrance. They eventually spotted Simon drive past in my Mondeo. As they were off-loading me, another ambulance driver from an adjacent vehicle dropped an implement, which they all joked about (it was all incoherent to me). On being wheeled into the entrance I remarked: "You're all so happy!"

Once inside, they booked me into "Casualty", but there were no cubicles available, so I had to wait on the stretcher in an adjacent corridor. The ambulancemen waited with me (fortunately!) but only because they needed the stretcher apparently!

A little while later I was pleased to look up and see Simon had arrived, chatting to the ambulancemen. I didn't notice his arrival so I had no idea of how long he had been there. The passage of time didn't seem to bother me as much as it usually does when I'm left waiting anywhere.

Eventually, a young female doctor with long, dark hair, approached me, asking what had happened. I explained everything all over again and was wheeled into a large cubicle, accompanied by Simon and the ambulancemen, who told me how to manoeuvre onto the trolley bed, so they could have their stretcher back! They left with it, leaving Simon with me and the doctor, who then closed the curtains.

She continued to question me whilst I was being wired into a colourful monitor and had my blood pressure taken.....continually.....for five hours. It went up to 127 at one point, then back down to 112, then 103 – constantly fluctuating. I was beginning to speak more normally now. The doctor pricked my finger for blood – even though the paramedics had done so earlier. She then took a blood sample from my Hickman line for tests and promptly vanished.

I told Simon I was worried about letting Nick know where we were – when we left home to go shopping we told him we wouldn't be long! Simon managed to obtain a special phone from a blonde female nurse. He tried to ring Nick but only got his messaging service. Due to his suspected tonsilitis and glandular fever, we assumed he was possibly sleeping, as his illness had made him tired of late. However, we later discovered that he had been next door, shooting a rat in their garage!

Some time later a blonde female nurse came in. I asked her about the blood test results and the whereabouts of the previous doctor, to which she replied that she was in a meeting doing a "handover" session and there were no results as yet.

The nurse asked me what had happened, so I told her. She hooked me up to a fluid solution on a drip via my Hickman line and promptly vanished!

Some time later, a blonde male nurse came in. He asked the usual questions, entering my answers on his form. Then he asked if I knew where I was. I thought that was a silly question and incredulously replied "In <u>hospital!</u>"

He then asked if I knew which town, so I told him. He explained that they have to check these things because I had collapsed.

He then put my forefinger in a grey, peg-shaped piece of plastic to test my pulse – something to do with my oxygen levels. There was a bright red light inside. I kept this on for the duration, studying my monitor. He promptly vanished like the others!

I was getting uncomfortable lying down, so I sat up – for the next five hours!

Simon sat next to my bed, occasionally leaving to feed the car park machines, who were their usual hungry selves! At one point he actually nodded off!

Some time later a small, young, balding man came in with a machine to take my ECG. He had to remove my tights in order to place the little square papers (with round bits on) on my lower shins. I removed my jumper so he could place more under my breasts (what was left of them), on my shoulders, at my waist and almost everywhere! He covered most of my body with a long, green gown. He told me to keep very still. The results were instant but he told me I had to wait for another nurse to reveal them to me later because he wasn't allowed to. Then, guess what, he promptly vanished!

Later (around 6 pm), a Senior Registrar came in to tell me the general results. Apparently I had no dehydration (due to the fluid line), my glucose level was OK and my pulse was now OK. *However*, I was anaemic and my blood pressure was quite low. I asked what caused this and what to do if it happened again, hopefully in a less embarrassing place! He informed me that the chemicals in my body (the chemotherapy ones) were obviously playing havoc with my systems. If it happens again, all I could do would be to lie down to get the blood back up to my head.

I told him how I had felt, explaining that a similar thing nearly occurred at home the previous evening, during dinner, when I suddenly felt giddy and tired and had to lie down on my bed. I remarked that I was annoyed at having to miss my Writers' Circle Christmas meal the previous Tuesday due to extreme tiredness and asked him what I should do about the forthcoming meals – one with my drama group and the other with Simon's employer. He replied that if I felt faint again, just to lie down! I wasn't particularly keen on going horizontal in front of Simon's workmates, let alone possibly vomiting again! Embarrassing or what!

Then he followed suit and vanished.

Later, the ECG man came back with the ECG specialist, who said that everything was not too bad, barring my low blood pressure. They now just needed to test my ECG whilst I stood up. I asked if the floor was cold, as I had nothing on my feet. However, I needn't have worried as it was quite warm.

The two men each held onto one of my arms as I was standing, then let go. I was OK for this test but was relieved to sit down again on the edge of the bed. The ECG man asked if I felt alright to go home. I said yes. He therefore suggested that Simon took me to our car by wheelchair then, guess what, they all vanished!

Simon came back a little later, pushing a brown, leather wheelchair into the cubicle. I took some of the hospital's small, grey "sick trays" with me (I wasn't taking any chances!). I carefully placed myself on it and he wheeled me through several corridors to the exit, leaving me for a few moments whilst he went to get the car. I waited for my ride home in the near-empty foyer until he returned and carefully helped me into the passenger seat before returning the wheelchair to its base in the foyer.

After about 12 miles, I began feeling sick again. I was glad I had the "sick trays" in the car with me, as I duly vomited once we were about half a mile from home (I just couldn't contain it any longer). I thought it just had to be <u>my</u> car I was in and not his! Suddenly, I had trouble catching my breath whilst vomiting. Simon told me to breathe slowly. It gradually subsided. He stopped the car by the roadside so that I could empty the contents into the kerb. I felt too ill to feel guilty at the time. I arrived shattered and drawn and went straight to bed.

CHAPTER TWENTY-TWO

Christmas

The following day Nick had difficulty swallowing and consequently couldn't eat or drink anything. To cut a long story short, Simon had to admit him to hospital the next day, to see a specialist. He remained there for the next few days.

I had to miss my drama group's annual Christmas meal that evening, which, coincidentally, took place at the same venue as the Writers' group meal. I was much too tired to attend (I had to be – I wouldn't normally forego having a nice meal with friends!)

Sunday, 7/12/08: After deliberating for some time about whether or not to attend Simon's works "do", I eventually decided to go with him – after all, I had refrained from attending the previous evening's event, especially to give me time to recuperate as far as possible. I thought as long as I could be seated near the Ladies' loo, I'd be fine!

It was at a nice pub/restaurant off the beaten track, about three miles away. The event was due to commence at 7.30 and Simon and I were the first to arrive, to be met by the managers who had organised it. It was a cold night but inside it was lovely and warm; with Christmas decorations everywhere. The tables were set in a very large square to accommodate the 20-odd staff members and their partners. One or two of the store managers kindly asked how I was doing – they were all aware of my "condition". We all had a lavish three-course meal. Later, Simon and I won a raffle prize – a large box of shortbread biscuits, naturally being the product produced by his employer! The evening ended with a quiz, during which I actually managed to get a couple of answers correct! We went home at about 10.30.

8/12/08:   Simon's 51st birthday! Unfortunately, Nick was still in hospital, on a drip.

We had a few visitors at our house that day: Dave (from Drama), Alan and even our Avon lady, Karen. Unfortunately, most of them missed Simon because he was still at work and didn't finish until 8 pm!

During the day, I arranged to have a nice big bunch of flowers sent to the staff and customers at the café, via Interflora. The card read something like "To the staff and customers at Bay Tree Café...who were very kind and helpful to me in my hour of need on Friday, 5th December. With grateful thanks," then my name. I paid £20 (which I couldn't really afford, but it was worth it) and, on discussing with the shop assistant why I was sending them, I discovered that she, too, had contracted breast cancer some years ago! This made her very sympathetic, especially when I explained what had happened that day!

Simon and I drove to hospital to pick Nick up from hospital as he was apparently a lot better now.

9/12/08: We took Nick to see one of our surgery's GPs, who advised that she thought he had, indeed, contracted glandular fever, explaining why the long, dangly thing (I always forget its correct name – sounds something like a sarcophogus!) at the back of his throat had swollen.

11/12/08:   Had Gill over for lunch. Before that I had to pick up the rest of Nick's prescription.

12/12/08:   10.45: The District Nurse visited as usual. Five minutes later, Brenda and Alan arrived from Berkshire, dropping off Simon's mum and dad at our house to stay for the weekend. Coincidentally, Christine and Alan had also invited Simon and I for dinner, so we postponed that to another day.

After refreshments, Brenda and Alan went on to visit Brenda's sister in Somerset.

13/12/08:   I noticed it was painful to pass urine. I rang the hospital who advised that it was very probable that I had a urine infection, whereby even flushing with water wouldn't help, and the pain would only get much worse if left untreated. Therefore they suggested I go to my local "Minor Injuries" hospital urgently, to be seen by a doctor, rather than a nurse, as it was only two weeks since I had finished chemotherapy. Then I waited for the local county doctors special telephone line to get back to me after I had explained the situation. When they finally did, they advised the same.

I apologised to Simon's parents that I had to drag their son away to escort me to the local hospital but they insisted this was much more important and that I should deal with it immediately. I left them both watching TV as Simon drove me a mile away to the hospital (at least it was nearer than the main hospital).

Whilst sitting in the waiting room, I found myself reading the "New Scientist" magazine, as you do! (No "Hello" magazines in *this* hospital!) I was particularly interested to read the health section which was discussing migraines. I had been having some myself for the past year, having never had any previously. The article stated that these could sometimes be an indication of the brain condition leading to neurological disease. Oh great, I thought! Now I was going mad!

After supplying a urine sample, the nurses there confirmed I did have an infection and supplied me with antibiotics to take for a week to get rid of it.

14/12/08   Simon, his parents, Nick and I all had lunch at the same pub/restaurant at which we had recently had his Marks and Sparks Christmas meal. It was very busy that day but nonetheless enjoyable. I went with Simon's dad to the carvery section, whilst the others waited at the table. His dad and I are the slowest eaters, so I thought it best we served ourselves first! We queued a few minutes before it was our turn. His dad obtained the meat on his plate first then went on to the vegetables, whilst I acquired my meat. By the time I caught up with him, I noticed he was attempting to pour custard onto his plate of roast beef and had to quickly prevent this by showing him where the gravy was! (Well, he was 91 and a little frail – though still with the general looks and demeanour of a grand gentleman who was very popular with his peers at Henley Golf Club!)

15/12/08: In the morning, I was able to drive Simon's parents to a rendezvous some 15 miles away, where they could pick up a lift for the remaining 115 miles from Brenda and Alan. Nick was with me. After bidding a fond farewell to them all, he and I stayed for lunch at the Little Chef (which was the rendezvous point), then I took him for another driving lesson in my car on some private land near where we live.

16/12/08: At 11 am, I had a pre-arranged visit at our house by Gina from Hospiscare, together wth a young, male medical student. I gave her a Christmas card meant for all the staff and we chatted over a cup of tea (we all had one!) about my condition and it was nice to hear Gina's comments about how Simon "looked very caring" and that I was "coping brilliantly". Everyone was always saying that, but I'm sure the "brilliance factor" must be greater for those who are surviving and coping with more terminal conditions. They're the ones who are coping "brilliantly"; it's easier to cope if there's a chance, no matter how small, of surviving than if you're told your illness is terminal. Still, it didn't hurt to hear it, I suppose.

17/12/08: Nick attended the doctor's for "Open Access Surgery", which isn't as bad as it sounds – it was just the name for waiting in the surgery, taking your turn to have another blood test, rather than a pre-arranged appointment system.

18/12/08: Last posting date for second class letters! Yes, I still had to get on with my life, including Christmas arrangements!

At 9 am Simon attended the local Physiotherapist's department for his neck and "tennis elbow" problem. (This wasn't a very healthy year for our family!)

In the evening, I accompanied Simon to one of the farms where he did some shooting, in order for him to drop off their Christmas presents – his usual bottle of whisky (or port - it's usually something of that ilk) and Stilton cheese. The farmer, Peter, and his wife, Janet, kindly invited us into their large house and we sat in the lounge, drinking coffee, being warmed by the log burner taking pride of place at the back of the room. Their large Alsation dog was very friendly and eventually fell asleep near the fire (I guess we bored him). I discovered they, like ourselves, weren't native to this part of the country, settling about 15 years ago after leaving the home counties, as apparently, (as I had discovered in my two years here) had many residents in this area.

19/12/08:   The District Nurse came in the morning, as usual. Zoe popped round at 1 pm and stayed a while. Then Simon and I had our massages by Caroline at 5.30 and 6.30 respectively. It was very relaxing, listening to the soft, instrumental music, despite the obvious problem she was having with the cassette in the machine, which kept "jumping", disturbing the transquil flow of music!

20/12/08:   Last posting date for first class letters! I'd posted all my cards by now (I hoped!).

21/12/08:   Well, Christmas was nearly here – my first Christmas with cancer. At least I didn't have to contend with chemo; I was able to enjoy the time of year without vomiting and yet I felt sorry for everyone who wasn't as fortunate and had to remain in hospital for this lovely time of the year.

7pm, our immediate neighbours either side of us came round, as arranged, for sherry and mince pies (as they did every year), as did Christine and Alan. None of them came empty handed, so there was plenty of food and refreshment to go round, if you know what I mean! We had an enjoyable evening (at least, I hope they did!)

22/12/08:   The day had come to have my "plumbing" removed. I arrived at the hospital shortly before 11 am. Simon and I handed over a large box of Roses chocolates and a Christmas card for all the staff (chemo and oncology), signed "Vomit Woman"!

I was taken to one of the beds in the far corner of the chemo treatment room, where the curtains were pulled round to provide a little dignity as I changed into their usual "half-gowns". I was asked if I minded that a student nurse remove my Hickman line, under the supervision of a doctor. I didn't mind – not for this minor op. I was originally led to believe it would be a fairly straight-forward procedure, however, it took longer than I expected. Simon waited in the main waiting room (the one with the large fish tank!), whilst the student did his best to pull the long, white tube through a little cut he had made at the top of my chest. He had to struggle somewhat when it came to manoeuvring the "cuff" out, so the doctor advised slicing me up a bit more to facilitate removal of the square, white, plastic box-shaped thing. At one point, they were both pressing down on that part of my chest (to stop me bursting open?) whilst the student gradually eased the long tube from inside me. After about an hour I was free!

24/12/08:   Christmas Eve: I picked Simon up from work at 8 pm then he and I popped into André's and Brian's places with bottles of wine and cards. (Brian was Simon's former employer before he worked for M & S.) We celebrated Christmas for a couple of hours with them and other friends, before going on to Midnight Mass and Holy Communion at St Paul's Church. We always try to attend a local church to celebrate Christmas – probably trying to salve our consciences for not attending any other time?

25/12/08:   After all the previous week's celebrations, we had a nice, quiet, family Christmas at home, just me, Simon and Nick. It was lovely. Simon helped me prepare the dinner (roast turkey, yum! - I'd love to be a vegetarian but poultry just tastes too nice – especially as I was no longer being sick!) We also had plenty to drink, and lots of boxes of chocolates had been provided by friends! I was so grateful I could really appreciate this time of the year without being severely ill.

27/12/08:   Picked Nick and a couple of his friends up from the local train station (they had been to the city centre that day).

29/12/08: Speaking on the phone to my friend Irene. Her husband, John, was recovering from a back operation. We discussed my not looking forward to the mastectomy, which was fairly imminent. As my friend Ada had mentioned, when we bashed into each other recently at

Tesco's, at least it will be behind me, I related to Irene. "Well, the event, not the boob!" I clarified. She made some remark about a pantomime, along the context of me being a writer, I presumed! But I thought better of it and decided to turn the experience into a book, rather than a pantomime, albeit having a close resemblance to such!

CHAPTER TWENTY-THREE

New Year, New Problems

For a change, we celebrated the New Year somewhat quietly. We "saw it in" by watching events on the TV – I suppose we'd had enough excitement in the past year.

I had just enough hair on the top of my head to comb now!

2/1/09: Christine kindly invited us over for dinner with her and Alan at their dairy farm, as the event had been postponed when Simon's parents visited us. I wasn't confident enough to go without my wig but we had a lovely time – We arrived at 6.30. Dinner was followed by a game of pool in the pool room, then card games like whist in the lounge, sitting on comfy armchairs in front of the largest open fire you can imagine! We left around 11 pm. Unfortunately, due to their ever-nearer moving date (ironically, to a house with the same number as ours!), our days of enjoyable evenings in their abode would be short now! The property is rented and Alan's virtually retired now; even the herd of cows had gone (sold, not vanished!). Still, at least our friends will be nearer to us!

3/1/09: Janet and Peter popped round to give us a huge joint of beef from their farm (as a "thank you" for the presents we gave them at Christmas, which they must have enjoyed!)

5/1/09: Thoughts were turning to my drama group's next production, Agatha Christie, and a Stage Production Meeting was consequently held at Jerry's house with the stage crew. I wasn't needed.

6/1/09: Whilst walking along the high street in our local town with

Nick, on the way to his bank, he was suddenly accosted by a tall, young girl of his age, who went right up to him, hugged him in a familiar way and said, unashamedly, "Hello gorgeous!" before going on her way. I may as well not have been there! Nick and I continued to the bank and I naturally had to ask who the girl was. He said, nonchalantly, that he knew her but didn't know her name (though he later admitted it might have been Naomi!). That was so typical of him – he hardly knows any names of the girls he knows! He's always getting cards and little presents from girls, ever since he was, well, almost a toddler! Brenda's sister told us at a social function once that, due to Nick's striking good looks, he's going to break a lot of hearts! Actually, I remember a Sainsbury checkout lady saying the same thing when he was a toddler in a push-chair – he's always been good-looking. Takes after his father, but don't tell him that: he'll get a big head!

4 pm: I had a massage performed by Caroline.

7/1/09: All Woolworths stores have gone bust now. So, too, have most of the Marks and Spencer Simply Food chain. We learned today that Simon will be made redundant in three months' time – just what we needed – (not). The recession was finally taking hold. Would we be able to pay the mortgage if he couldn't find any work? I was in no fit state to return to work yet. Guess it was up to Nick to keep us afloat for now!

8/1/09: 11.40: I dropped Simon off at work, arranging to pick him up at 7.55, which entailed waiting in a large, empty, dark public car park out of sight of his firm.

But until then, I met up with Ann from my old solicitors' firm in town. She was a young-looking 60, always immaculately dressed, as befitting a solicitor's receptionist. We both had a love of amateur theatrics – she was a singer in a musical society at her home town some twelve miles away. (I can't sing for toffee – except in the bathroom when I think no-one can hear me! My friend Heather and I once auditioned for Hughie Green's TV show "Opportunity Knocks" when we were about 15, calling ourselves "Sapphire" but, needless to say, got nowhere!). I saw a few of my colleagues at the office who all said how well I looked (well, I <u>was</u> wearing a wig!). Ann and I then went for lunch to a local, quaint café (not the one where I had fainted – that was a different town) situated at the rear of an antique shop in the high street. It was rather small but interestingly decorated with large black and white, wall-sized photographs, depicting 19th century ladies and gents on small river boats. The two window-sills displayed unusual antiques for sale – brass kettles, funny shaped candlabras and small statues. Beyond that you could see part of the garden area with white plaster-cast statues raised on 12 inch square boards displayed on the garden fence. We didn't wait too long for lunch (which was handy for Ann, who only had an hour before she had to return to work). We chatted about old times and she also related the sad details of her ninety-year-old mother's fairly recent death. After lunch we took a brisk walk back to her office, then I returned to my car and drove home.

CHAPTER TWENTY-FOUR

Everyone thinks I'm brave, but I'm not....

9/1/09: 11 am: Nick had to have yet another blood test at the surgery to test for glandular fever again.

3 pm: I had to attend a postponed "interview" at the local Job Centre regarding any benefits I was obtaining. It was short and pleasant, which was more than I could say for the long and painful process of trying to get any benefits, half of which I wasn't entitled to simply because I was married! Obviously working all my life since 16, paying income tax and national insurance for 34 years, counts for very little. Oh, but apparently I was entitled to Council Tax benefit.......of 97p! That really helped my financial situation!! I told Simon I'd be much better off (financially) if I divorced him, slept with lots of men and had lots of babies, demanding somewhere to live –then I'd be entitled to more financial aid! End of political speech.

Because I now had a little tuft of dark grey hair on top of my head, my new nickname from Simon (don't ask what my old one was) was Tufty! Or sometimes Tintin - except my hair was the wrong colour!

11/1/09: Nick turned 17. I couldn't believe how old he was getting – he'd soon be a man (as opposed to a boy, not a woman!). I treated him to a meal with Simon at the same restaurant Simon had had his works "do". I told him this was probably the last time I'd be able to spend on him like this due to the money situation, so I suggested he lap it up while he could.

12/1/09: Around 8.30 am. It was a dismally rainy day (of which we've had many lately). As Simon wasn't due to start work until 11.45, he drove Nick about ten miles to a bus station where he was meant to be picked up by a training company van (to take him to a company where he could train as a plasterer/dry liner, although he would really have made a better electrician or carpenter). Some time after they left home, I answered a telephone call from Nick to say they hadn't been picked up. So I rang the manager of the company, who said a couple of other boys had also been missed, so he asked if Simon could take Nick all the way there himself (an extra 7 miles or so) but I had to inform him he didn't know the way. To cut a (long) story short, they came back a little while later, both looking like drowned rats due to standing waiting in the rain for the van which, we later learned, had been parked in a different place to where we had been told. I don't think Nick was meant to do that course, so he cancelled it anyway, as he wasn't really that keen.

13/1/09:   Gill paid for us both to have lunch at the local inn. I learned that she was, in fact, a distant relative of the distinguished actor Sir Michael Redgrave! She often comments (as if to prove it?) that she has the "Redgrave nose"! My only claim to fame was that I had performed in a theatrical competition at the Redgrave Theatre in Farnham, Surrey! Our play won! It was a spoof of "The Blob"! (Well, the theatre was named after Sir Michael, that's some connection!)

At one point we found ourselves discussing "women's things", amongst which was the fact that I often got very hot, then quickly cooled down. She told me it sounded "menopausal" and usually started at the neck/chest, making its way to the head. She added that drinking alcohol often prompts it. I was on Southern Comfort and lemonade at the time! She said I had "bed sweats" to look forward to next. Charming! Couldn't wait!

We went back to my house for coffee. She left around 4 pm.

15/1/09:   I got a letter from the hospital to advise me of a meeting I was to attend on the 20th to "discuss results". It would probably also confirm that the surgeon would lop my breast off!

Later that day Nick was discussing parents, particularly who he preferred to take him for driving lessons. Instead of his usual insults he throws at me, he commented on the fact that I "don't moan, am fun and like 21st century music!" *(Sorry Simon. He he!)*

16/1/09: I used my meagre savings to purchase Simon a gold wedding band. It was something I had always wanted him to wear but, because he was predominantly in the building trade, he thought it inadvisable in case it got damaged. Of course, he was no longer in the building trade now so I thought this was a good opportunity to get him one. I don't know....I just felt like I particularly wanted him to wear something significant now as a reminder of me...maybe....just in case, but I never put it quite like that while we were choosing one – which turned out to be too big anyway – just my luck! He'd never worn any jewellery before, apart from a watch, and consequently, kept telling me how it felt like he was wearing a plaster on his finger! At one point, he threw a biscuit to Toby but the ring flew off his finger – it was obviously too loose! Needless to say he didn't wear it for long after that. Oh well...I tried...

Whilst in town, I also paid £3 in a cancer charity shop (naturally!) for a hessian-style shopping bag with large, pink flowers on it, saying *"Together We Will Beat Cancer – Cancer Research UK"*. I said to the shop assistant, as I was handing over the money, "Most people know I've got it anyway – so I may as well advertise the fact!"

Later that day I saw a televisions programme talking about breast implants causing pain and problems....I thought I would probably experience that, knowing my luck, so I concluded that, if there was no other way of replacing the lost boob, I would therefore probably only have one breast the rest of my life after the mastectomy. I related my apprehension concerning the op to Simon, who responded by stating, in a matter-of-fact fashion, that it was better to lose a boob than your life!

17/1/09: 10.30: It was Nick's first official driving lesson today, until midday. At 12.30 he came with me to take Toby to a dog-grooming shop in one of the town's back streets. It only cost £25, so I raided my savings again to treat our dog, in case both he and I never got the chance again. Because he was quite old now (13 ½), he had to be lifted by the scruff of his neck and the other end, in order to get in and out of the car, hence I required Nick's help!

We picked Toby up at 2.30 to see he had been nicely cleaned up/ washed and had his nails trimmed (I could actually see the fur-less nails now!).

19/1/09:   Gill picked me up at 7.15 for our drama group's Committee Meeting held at Jerry's house. We had a lively debate, mostly about the forthcoming Agatha Christie production, as well as future venues (our town doesn't have a proper theatre....scratch that. Our town doesn't have a theatre at all. Full stop!).

Christine rang to ask if I was going to the hospital on my own the next day. I said I would be fine as it had been a while since I had finished my chemo and had the "fainting" episode! But it was nice of her to ask.

CHAPTER TWENTY-FIVE

It's A Funny Shape Anyway!

20/1/09:   I was writing a list of what to take to hospital for my op, when Nick saw it and piped up: "spare boob"!

I thought I was getting brave today, as I popped next door to Barbara and George to return the books they kindly loaned me last year, without wearing my wig!

Every now and again, when alone in the house, my mind would wander to the forthcoming events. I often wondered how on earth aethiests and agnostics survived such ordeals. I found myself glancing at the framed image of Christ on our mantlepiece – I bought it from Exeter Cathedral many years ago when we first visited Devon. Whenever I had the opportunity, I would mention to anyone who listened that the outcome of my condition ultimately depended on a "higher" being. OK, so the NHS was obviously playing a big part and I'm very grateful for that, of course. And cancer treatments are improving all the time. But....ultimately....I just had to have faith because, well, when all is said and done, it's really out of our hands....isn't it?.....And, like my mum and her mum before her always used to say: "what's to be will be...."

Gina, from Hospiscare, rang to enquire, as Christine did, about my travelling alone to hospital today. Again I confirmed I should be OK in this instance but thanked her for asking. I added that, actually, I was looking forward to listening to my own choice of music in the car and, anyway, I already knew the outcome of the meeting – I would have to have a mastectomy, so I didn't really know why the meeting was so necessary; they had never seemed able to advise me on how my chemo was doing on the cancer, which is what I really wanted to know.

It took me about 20 minutes to drive to the hospital for my 2.25 appointment. Unfortunately, as was usual for that time of day (or almost any time of day there really!), I had a great deal of trouble trying to find a parking space. There wasn't one space in the five large car parks. That's right – not one space. Cars were queuing everywhere in the vain hope someone would vacate a space for them! I even tried parking in the surrounding streets and thought I had found a space, only to discover it was for residents parking only! In all, I drove around the hospital and the streets about five or six times – passing each time, as I did, the same man standing at the hospital bus stop – he must have wondered what on earth I was doing because I was still driving round in circles 45 minutest later! A record by all accounts! A couple of times I had to use my mobile phone to let the department know I was in the vicinity but still in my car, unable to park! Finally, during my last call to them, I suddenly spotted a car moving out of a space just as another vehicle had started to enter that car park. I called into the phone: "Sorry – I've got to go! There's a space! Bye!" and sped off the few yards into the vacated space just before the incoming car saw it! Phew! What a relief! Then I had to enter the closest department, which happened to be the chemo department, to explain my dilemma in parking so I could get a ticket for that particular car park because it was really only for patients actually having chemo that day, so they graciously gave me a permit for 20p before I rushed along the corridor then up the stairs and along the next corridor until I finally arrived at the reception and waiting area of the Surgical Outpatients. The receptionist completely understood my situation, having received a message – everyone there knew only too well of the parking problems that the hospital had.

There were quite a few people already in the waiting room. After waiting about 45 minutes to be seen, I was shown into a room to discuss my forthcoming mastectomy with Mr Ferguson and Annie, one of the Breast Care nurses. Annie was very friendly and understanding, as all of the Breast Care nurses seemed to be. She had long, dark hair and a bubbly personality – a bit like me....before I got cancer.

I was given the date of the operation: Friday, 30th January – a day that will go down in "infamy" in my books (including this one!). I resigned myself to the inevitable, stating: "Oh well, it's a funny shape anyway..."

I could tell they wanted to laugh but tried to do it sympathetically! I added that I realised it was better to have the lumpectomy first, creating a strange shape of the breast, because then, by the time it comes to have the full mastectomy, one isn't so disturbed about the removal, due to its weird shape – you might as well have nothing there, as a funny shaped breast with a lump missing!

We arranged for me to have another "Pre-Op Assessment" the following week, where Annie could also discuss the procedure in more detail, as well as show me photographs of other women's ops plus reconstructive photographs.

The subject of this book arose at one point, and I was expressing my concern at being able to find alternative names for the real people in order to preserve their privacy and make them anonymous - didn't want to offend anyone. (What's that? – Too late now?!) So if you see any references here to "Posh and Becks" or "Brad and Angelina", you'll know they're really Mr Ferguson and Annie (Annie's suggestions! – Thanks Annie!)

So I said goodbye to Posh and Becks who gave me some paperwork to go and have a blood test and ECG on the ground floor, several long corridors away. It was now 5 o'clock. Unfortunately, though I was in time for the ECG, the haematology department was closed, so I trundled back to the now quiet Surgical Outpatients reception to let them know that I would be available to have it done a couple of days before the op anyway. The receptionist said she would pass the message on.

The next day, I was just about to drive to pick Simon up from work when I got a call from Don of the Writers' Circle. He asked how I was doing and kindly offered to give me a lift to hospital if ever I needed it, adding that it would be no problem especially as he had to make fairly frequent trips there himself anyway. I thanked him for the offer, saying I may just take him up on it some time.

Simon's mum also rang during the day to advise that our home town had apparently been on the television in the programme "Bargain

Hunt", where they particularly showed the antiques shops which lined the high street.

On the news it was stated that there were now 1.92 million people in the U.K. who were unemployed (so Simon would be in good company!).

I found myself watching the programme on TV documenting and serialising Jade Goody's fight against cervical cancer (the ex- "Big Brother" celebrity). She had been told she had only months to live. From what I could tell on the TV documentary, her situation was far, far worse than mine and she was only 27. I was just glad I had at least always had cervical smears to detect just such a condition. I always seemed to be aware of other people being afflicted with cancer, much more than before, and felt particularly sorry for anyone contracting it at a young age, especially children. I couldn't imagine the psychological effect such news would have on youngsters, who had barely begun their lives, or their families.

It was interesting to hear her comments that, on receiving the news, she was neither depressed nor angry – she would just "get on with her life". And that was exactly my attitude. I was more annoyed about how slow my laptop was at the time whilst trying to write this book!

Why be depressed and, particularly, why be angry? Who can you vent your anger against? Who can you blame? No-one. It's just tough – you've just got to get on with it. So that's what I was doing....and Lord knows I always had plenty to be getting on with – still have, as I write this. There just never seems to be enough time....

CHAPTER TWENTY-SIX

Paws for Thought

23/1/09:   Nick had his second "official" driving lesson today. Apparently he got on very well.

5.30 pm: Simon had his massage from Sue, as Caroline was on holiday. It seemed to do him good, as they usually do.

Had a phone call from mum – we spoke about the forthcoming operation and she told me I was "bubbly and positive" and said she would pray for me. I needed that. I told her that it would only be a two hour op (the reconstructive one is five hours), one hour of which was with the anaesthetist and one hour in "recovery".

Sharyl also rang and we discussed implants. She suggested I make enquiries about "immune suppressants", such as they give to transplant patients, to fool the body into thinking material entering the body is not "foreign matter".

That weekend, Simon drove me and Toby to the nearest beach and left us there. No, sorry, I mean took us there so we could all have a few hours break from the current rigours of life. It was a rather pebbly beach, near a busy town. It was a fairly wet, blustery day and we should really have stayed at home but I just wanted a day out before the "big day", so Simon kindly obliged. Toby was also due for a good day out too, although it nearly didn't end that way....

Despite the time of year the town was quite busy, mostly with families and young children. We English don't get put off by a little bit of bad weather! Once on the beach, we let Toby off the lead. A middle-aged lady with her own, large dog ambled by, watching Toby's antics as Simon continually threw stones in the sea for him to catch. Unfortunately, the sea was very rough; you could see a lot of 'white horses', and the tide kept rushing in relentlessly, sweeping Toby off his wobbly paws more than once (well, he wasn't only ill, he was nearly 14 years old, not a young pup any more). He managed to regain his posture nearly every time but I was getting worried. I called to Simon, asking if he would be able to swim after Toby if he got swept out to sea, because I could see that was where events were heading! Simon continued to throw stones to him, but edging them towards the windbreaker nearer to the promenade. But it was no good – after racing after each pebble, Toby still kept losing his balance with every rush of the tide, slipping under more than once. I was scared for him, even though he didn't seem to be bothered, surfacing moments later all the time, eagerly awaiting the next stone! But I was worried about the time he may not surface. Simon finally managed to grab him by the scruff of his neck, struggling to lift him away from the ever-present tide, before eventually dragging him along the beach and up the incline that led back to the promenade. I was never so relieved! We didn't stay too long after that. Especially as Toby's paw had obviously started to leak blood by the cancer tumour. You could follow his trail all around the increasingly empty town. (apologies to the council!) Poor dog. We took him home and bathed his paw. Ironically, he didn't seem any the worse for his experience! A couple of dog biscuits and he was happy as Larry!

Nick had more driving lessons the rest of the week – including a trip to the same town where Toby nearly drowned!

25/1/09:   Our home town was on the telly again, on "Bargain Hunt". It was the one time I was glad of TV repeats, enabling me to see what I had missed!

There were only three days left of me having two breasts. If I thought really hard about it, I felt sick to the stomach...when I actually tried to envisage it....so I stopped trying.

It cheered me up a little, the next day, when I received an email from BBC radio, quoting the sample they had read of my book as "readable and moving". Aah! (But I wasn't really going for "moving", I was going for "light hearted"!)

27/1/09:   My eyebrows were slowly returning – half of each had vanished during chemo and they were usually fairly thick and dark.

Gina, from Hospiscare, rang to check how I was doing. I told her that I was a little more apprehensive now that we were closer to the date of the mastectomy. She said she would ring again next Wednesday.

I tried to say to myself that they're "not removing my boob, they're (hopefully) removing the cancer".....

I felt a little more exhilarated when I was watching a woman at the end of a programme on TV (I seem to do that a lot, don't I?), who remarked with panache:

"There's a whole world out there – I feel I can do anything!" following a sci-fi programme stating that "they're human – they have spirit and are superior.."

It certainly lifted my spirit! Then I went back to typing this.

Nick came with me to take Toby to the vet. The dog groomer had told us that he could possibly have an infection due to bacteria getting into the wound as, when her face was near his paw whilst grooming him, she noticed a terrible smell coming from it. The vet suggested we use Hibiscrub solution to bathe it in, with painkilling tablets if he seemed to be in pain. He said antibiotics would only last about a week so it wouldn't be worthwhile having them. If he still seemed to be enjoying his quality of life, we should continue in that way, otherwise, he considered Toby too old for amputation of the toes, which would affect his balance.

I always felt quite sad about the fact that, there I was, being treated by the NHS for cancer, whilst poor Toby could only just wait for the inevitable, with minimum treatment.

CHAPTER TWENTY-SEVEN

A "Fresh of Breath Air"

28/1/09:   10.00 am: Pre-Op Assessment day at the hospital. A busy day, by all accounts, where everything was discussed and examined!

I had to park in the street due to no available spaces in the hospital car parks. I was only allowed three hours there, so I kept my fingers crossed that I wouldn't be too long (huh!).

My first port of call (of many, I might add) was the Parkerswell Ward, where I was promptly handed a note written by Annie asking me to go to the Breast Care Unit, Area F Level 2 after completing my pre-op checks. A young auxilliary nurse with short, dark hair, introduced herself and pointed out a waiting area where I was to return after having tests, before directing me through to Medical Outpatients where I was to have a blood test, then ECG. I sat, each time, in the waiting area (actually a narrow corridor!), along with half a dozen other patients on a neat little row of chairs outside the departments. The person on the chair nearest the door was always meant to be the next patient to be seen, so every time they were called, the rest of us patients had to each move up a chair, in order to be nearer the door and eventually next in the queue – it was like "musical chairs"! But the occasional commotion gave us all a much needed laugh! (us English, again – nothing gets us down!)

Eventually I was next to be seen. The chair in the haemotology section was extremely comfortable, so much so that I almost regretted having to leave, but I didn't really want to have any more blood taken from me so I went on to have my ECG. The nurse "wired me up" – fortunately I had "pop sox" under my trousers, so I didn't have to remove my trousers to facilitate wires being attached to my legs. They went everywhere – shoulders, back, chest, under my boobs, stomach, sides of the waist, thighs, shins, you name it! The nurse looked at the monitor for a few seconds while the results printed out, then removed the stickies attaching the wires (well, most of them – there always seemed to be one of two left lurking around that they missed!). As usual, she wasn't allowed to give me the results, so I wandered back to the waiting area I had originally been directed to, studying the graph she had given me, trying to make head or tail of it. The wiggly lines seemed fairly consistent and I hoped that was a good sign.

There was a dark-haired middle-aged lady sitting on one of few chairs in the waiting area where I placed myself. I later discovered her name was Mrs Smith. She was reading a magazine. Whilst waiting, Mr Ferguson and a nurse passed through the double doors and through the waiting area. He spotted me and called, en route to the other reception: "Hi! How are you?"

"Fine!" I smiled.

What a twit! Why on earth did I say that? How could I possibly be fine with what was in store for me in two days' time? Oh well.....

Shortly after, Annie appeared, said hello to me and began discussing medical things with the lady sitting next to me. From the (not very private) discussion they were having, it was obvious that the lady had never, even at this stage of events, seen her surgeon – who happened to be mine, Mr Ferguson!

Annie and I joked about how this lady really should see him! (And we weren't really referring to his medical capacity!) I would say more but he may read this one day (Ha!) or at least Simon might! (double Ha!)

Annie asked if I had received her note and I said I had. We arranged a time to meet, but I did warn her that it wouldn't be much longer before my car park time ran out. We decided to play it by ear.

A little while later the lady next to me was called to be seen (not by Mr Ferguson), leaving me on my own until another lady replaced her a few seats away. She was a nice, elderly lady and we chatted for a while, as you do.

Eventually it was my turn to be seen. The auxilliary nurse led me to a room where a registered nurse was sitting at a desk. She was in her thirties, with medium length blonde hair. Both she and the other nurse were very pleasant and made me feel relaxed, as did most of the staff. The registered nurse asked me a ton of questions about my medical history in order to complete the form in front of her. Questions like did I drink, smoke, my parents' health, other illnesses, bar breast related ones. I mentioned the fact that, after my last operation, I was naturally starving (due to having "nil by mouth" beforehand) and had to watch everyone eat their meals before I could have what was left on the food trolley as nothing had been ordered for me. The nurse told me to therefore order a meal for later as soon as I arrived for the operation. She also advised me to inform the anaesthetist about my vomiting problem (although I thought they would have all known about me by now!). Then the auxilliary nurse did the usual OBS, i.e. my blood pressure, height and weight (I hated having to face my weight!). I asked her to translate the results into pounds and ounces because their scales were always in kilos! In fact, the height was also metric but I know my height because it's always the same!

Then she asked me to do the "swabs" procedure, as I had done before, to check for MRSA or similar. She inserted the long chop-stick style stick into my mouth until it reached the back of my throat. However, the gentle tickling which resulted almost made me feel sick! I tried to explain this to them both, which was difficult considering I had a stick stuffed in my mouth. This made me giggle, as far as I could, which in turn, made the nurses titter somewhat. So the auxilliary nurse removed it and placed another one inside my nostril. This tickled as well. I told them it made me want to sneeze! The registered nurse offered me a tissue, which I took. I began laughing so much my eyes began to water. I made a lot of silly cracks about the procedure and it wasn't long before we were all in hysterics! When it was time to leave the registered nurse tried to tell me she thought I was a "breath of fresh air" but by this time she was so confused that it came out as a "fresh of breath air"! But I knew what she meant.

I was told to wait outside again until I was seen by a junior doctor. Not long after he appeared and led me to his little office, which was adjacent to the nurses' office, and told me to take a seat next to his desk. He fired questions at me in order to complete the form in front of him – they were virtually identical to the ones I had already been asked and I didn't mind telling him so, but I still had to answer them. A few minutes into this, there was a knock at the door and the nurse I had just seen entered. On spotting me, she told us that she and the other nurse had stitches from all the laughing! I apologised! She gave the doctor some files and left.

The doctor then asked me to sit down on the nearby bed and move my hands. I don't know why, but I instinctively began to reach for my jumper in order to raise it to exhibit my breasts – I was so used to showing them to medical staff! He was obviously embarrassed (as I said, he was only a *young* doctor) and explained that he just needed to press my finger tips! On seeing that I was not only slightly embarrassed as well, but also bewildered, he explained that this procedure was to ascertain how quickly the blood returned to my fingers, after turning white from the pressing. He then felt the top arches of both feet (must have had some reason!) and asked to see my tongue (afterwards!). It was reassuring to hear him follow every step with the words "good" or "perfect"! Then it was time to listen to my heartbeat and the poor fellow thought this could be achieved through my clothes, but to no avail. So I ended up lifting my jumper anyway! He placed the stethoscope on my chest to listen, instructing me to take a deep breath: "In...."

I did as instructed.

"...And again..." he continued.

Barely breathing, I complained: "You've got to say 'Out' first!"

He said 'Out' and I breathed out.

"In...."

I took a deep breath again and before I had the chance to fully inhale, along came the instruction to exhale again!

He then felt the blood vessel on my neck, which is apparently the one directly from the heart and, finally, he listened to my pulse, before sending me off to see Annie in the Breast Care Clinic.

So off I trundled along the many corridors and flights of stairs, announcing myself at the Breast Care Clinic reception on arrival. I sat down, looking apprehensively at my watch, aware that my car park time was due to expire momentarily. I wondered how long Annie would be but I didn't have to wait long. She soon appeared and said hello, to which I replied "Goodbye, I've got to move my car, the time's run out!" The three hours' allotted time had, indeed, expired. She understood and agreed to wait while I took the long walk to feed the machine again.

I strode briskly for about fifteen minutes to my car where the payment machine informed motorists that they could not remain at that spot after the expiry time. So I had to drive around again looking for another space and eventually found one in another street, where I paid for another two hours (I'd spent £4 in total so far), trusting I wouldn't have to move again. I marched swiftly back to the Breast Care Clinic, a little fitter than when I left!

Annie showed me into a nice little room, with magnolia painted walls, reminiscent of a small hotel lounge. There were four cream-coloured, leather armchairs around a circular, wooden coffee table, a long wall mirror reflected the scene at the far end, near a tall, white standard lamp. Near the door there stood a very large chest of drawers with leaflets displayed on the top and a wooden slatted concertina style "changing" screen stood in the opposite corner.

I made myself comfortable on one of the armchairs as Annie left to make me a cup of coffee (which I was very grateful for!). On her return, she proceeded to show me lots of large colour photos of breasts after a mastectomy as well as after reconstructive surgery (she understood I had requested this some time ago, which I had). I told her one of the leaflets I had been given a while back mentioned a possibility of using one's stomach to facilitate a new boob but I was put off by the fact that it mentioned that it would then be sore and make coughing or bending down painful after such an operation. However, she put my mind at ease by informing me (whilst trying not to laugh I think) that this would only be for an initial two or three months after the op – not forever! She quelled another concern of mine regarding implant rejection by my own body (especially the way my body is); she said that such rejection might not actually happen, as tissue transferred from the stomach to the breast area would obviously be my own tissue and not "foreign matter" as such, therefore reducing the risk of rejection. Well, that was a relief! I said I was actually seriously considering the "stomach" tissue transplant because, as well as getting a new boob, it would also mean (hopefully) having a smaller waist! She didn't stop herself laughing this time.

She asked if I had seen a prosthetic breast which, of course, I hadn't. How could I? So she pulled one out of a box, like carefully whipping a rabbit out of a hat, and passed it to me to fondle, I mean feel, I mean, examine! Well, it was so soft and "wobbly", I remarked "This is better than my good one!", making her laugh again (someone should put her in one of my audiences if I ever do 'stand up'!). I remarked on its weight – I was surprised that it was quite a hefty piece of material. She said they come in various weights, which I suppose made sense.

Then she showed me one of their "temporary" ones which you wear for the first six weeks or so, whilst the scar is healing, called a "cumfie". The beige coloured exterior cloth covered a type of thick cotton wool (kind of like the stuffing one finds in teddy bears!) and the whole thing was shaped just like a breast (without a nipple!). Apparently both types are inserted into "pockets" in the bra, another sample of which she produced from a box.

I was curious about what actually happens to the breast after surgery and she informed me that the tissue goes to the Pathology department for analysis. It's apparently kept in liquid in a jar until it's needed. Not much you can say about that. Well there is, but not here!

Annie asked if I was nervous about the operation. I replied no – only about what I would see afterwards! I was therefore grateful to have seen the photos which at least gave me some idea of what to expect.

She advised me to bring all my bras in on the day of the operation, in order to see if any of them would be suitable for prosthesis insertion, which I agreed to do.

We discussed funding, especially in light of the fact that Simon was soon to be made redundant (in two months) and Nick was currently looking for work having left school a while back and I, of course, had very little in the way of benefits (due mostly, I understand, to being married – but let's not dwell on that again....), and my savings were almost depleted. She therefore kindly gave me a MacMillan's form to complete to help towards transport costs (especially with three weeks' worth of daily trips for radiotherapy soon) and a mastectomy bra. I thanked her (probably too profusely) as she also gave me some magazines selling mastectomy lingerie and swimwear before I left.

Ironically, I now had some time left on the car parking meter, so I popped over to the Force centre and had some hot chocolate and biscuits (I was starving!). I understood one was entitled to do this, even if one had no appointment there, as such. You could even just pop over there to pass the time while waiting to be seen in the main hospital. It was a lovely place – just like a hotel – and you were always made to feel welcome. I just never realised these places existed – well, I suppose that was because I had never had cancer before. I donated some money in the charity box and visited the small library there where I read a book written by another cancer patient, detailing her experience. I hoped it wasn't too similar to mine as I didn't want people thinking I was copying her, which I wasn't. In fact, it was very interesting and humourous in parts. So....not like mine then!

Back in the reception area I arranged for Simon to have one of his massages there on Friday whilst I was having my op. because I knew he would be bored silly. Luckily, there had been a cancellation at 10.30 – quite a good time, I thought.

Whilst sitting on the barstool there, another cancer patient appeared. She was a mature lady who was very obviously a skinhead due to the treatment.

"You're brave," I remarked, sitting there with my thick, brown wig on my head.

"People have to take me as they find me," she replied, "It was my mindset from the beginning...There's only really been one bad incident," she continued to explain about the time she was in a large Tesco's store with her 14 year old son, where a woman stared at her head in disgust. So her son called to this other woman; "It's not catching – my mum's got cancer!""

"I moved away, embarrassed," she concluded.

"I'm only gradually getting brave," I said, "I forgot to put my wig on in the car once and also popped round to see my neighbours and couldn't be bothered to put it on just to go next door."

The Force volunteer was obviously astounded that the hair she could see on my head was a wig. Myself and the other patient commented on how hot it gets when you wear a wig, so it's uncomfortable to keep it on for too long.

We bade each other goodbye and I set off home.

Later that evening, I was telling Simon about all the things I would have to bring on the day of the operation, i.e. food, return the library book I had borrowed from Force, all my bras – "to cut in half", he quipped! My family is so sympathetic! I sternly corrected him; "No.... to see if any are suitable for prosthesis insertion....." He continued sniggering. He's like that! He loves me really. At least he says he does! I do wonder sometimes!

CHAPTER TWENTY-EIGHT

A Titillating Experience

29/1/09:   Received cards from mum and dad and Nicki with sentiments "Thinking of You" on them, which I thought was very nice and thoughtful.

I felt a bit better today regarding going in for the op. Obviously it did me some good seeing Annie yesterday, allaying my fears, as it were.

Later in the day I was duffing Nick up on the sofa (don't worry – it was just a "tickling" session – yes, in spite of his age and his constant insults to me, he still likes to be treated like a toddler sometimes, but don't tell his friends!). I mentioned that this was his last chance to be tickled because I would only have one boob tomorrow and he replied "That's why God gave you two! He gave you two of everything!"

"But what about your mouth?" I queried.

"Who loses their mouth?" he asked incredulously. I thought "You don't!" But he always seems to get the last word......

That night Simon and I had trouble getting to sleep (rare for us!). It was midnight and we were both still awake.

"It's hard to sleep, isn't it?" he commented quietly.

I agreed, although I was surprised that he was having trouble, after all, it was me who was going to have an operation, not him. And yet I found it somehow sweet that it was affecting him too – aahh!

30/1/09:   The big day had arrived. We arrived at the hospital at 8.30 am. I was starving (not allowed food after 7pm the previous night). It was raining. A cold front was forecast coming from Russia the next week. Still, it didn't affect me, being in hospital. At least something went my way!

There were eight other people in the waiting room, amongst whom I recognised Mrs Smith. I wondered if she had yet met Mr Ferguson, if not she probably would now! We exchanged polite "hellos" then she conversed with her other half and I nudged mine to remove his elbows from the arm of my chair!

At one point there weren't enough chairs for everyone to sit on and one of the spouses had to sit, cross-legged, on the floor next to his wife. He didn't seem to mind at all – fortunately he was quite a young, healthy-looking chap. But then one of the nurses was shocked when she entered and saw this and said he shouldn't have to do that - she would arrange for another seat to be brought in but he insisted this wasn't necessary, he was fine as he was! It was taken in good humour by everyone in the room.

I was eventually called into a small office by Mr Ferguson's female SHO, who explained the possible after-effects of the procedure, i.e. I would probably be bruised, there may be bleeding, infection, etc. (oh joy!) and I had to sign a consent form to say I understood all the horrible things that might happen to me, or else I could just change my mind at not have the operation at all!

I said "OK then – bye!"

She laughed. Well, sort of.

So I signed yet another form before she drew a very large arrow on my body pointing to the breast to be operated on.

"That will come off won't it?" I asked, "The arrow, I mean. I know the breast will!"

She smiled and confirmed it wasn't indelible ink!

I returned to the waiting room and sat next to Simon.

Shortly afterwards, we were led down the corridor, past the ward I was in for my op last year. The nurse thought she had lost me for a moment, when I stopped to look at it! We had a little giggle about that as she continued to lead us a few corridors away and into a nice, bright, six-bedded Abbey Ward which was fully occupied. I was pleasantly surprised to be taken to the bed in the far corner. It had a window with a nice view of trees and a very old building across the road – possibly the original hospital. Only one other bed had a window beside it. One of the patients, Rosie, had been looking out of the middle window and was returning to her bed next to mine. She was a similar age to myself, with medium-length brown hair and a pleasant smile. We bid each other hello.

Simon and I settled on a couple of chairs in my "area". I looked at my bed next to me. It was very modern. I was impressed – well, to begin with anyway. I tried to operate the mattress, which was obviously one that could be bent into all sorts of shapes. The remote control device had various shaped and coloured buttons on it. I thought I had pressed the correct one to operate the bed and then a young student nurse called Amanda suddenly appeared from the nurses' station. Apparently I had called for a nurse instead! Fortunately she took it in good humour. We got on rather well for the duration – at least I think we did, don't know if she would agree!

I noticed all the beds had identification labels above the headboards, ranging from C1 to C6. Trust mine to have been "C4" – talk about explosive! *(for those of you who don't watch sci-fi films, C4's an explosive!)*

At 9.30 a female physiotherapist came along and gave me a leaflet to explain the different exercises I would need to carry out at various stages after the op. She showed me one or two of them, asking me to copy her. It was very straight-forward. However, as I explained to her, I did always feel silly doing the one where you stand up against a wall and reach out with your arm, making your fingers "walk" up and down the wall! OK if no-one was watching, I suppose.

Half an hour later another of Mr Ferguson's SHO's tried to take blood from me, saying it was in case I needed a blood transfusion. However, I had to tell her that blood had already been taken on Wednesday, two days earlier! She said she would need to take a blood test after the op. to check I hadn't lost too much blood.

10.30: Simon went for the massage I had booked for him, taking with him the book I had borrowed to be returned, leaving me to wait for my op.

11.45: I was bored now. I found myself constantly looking at my watch. I wondered when Simon would be back; he must have had his massage by now – I knew it was a long walk away though, past the many car parks! I stared out of the window again, admiring the views. Maybe I would catch a glimpse of Simon. Then I remembered the larger window near to mine, in the middle of the wall, between my bed and the bed opposite. This was where Rosie had been earlier. So I decided to admire the view from there, negotiating a table, linen trolley and drip stand, which were all in the way. On the way back, I forgot about the obstacle course and accidentally bashed into the drip stand, causing it to make a "clanging" noise. I hoped it didn't wake any of the sleeping patients. Amanda saw me from a distance, trying to straighten the device, and laughed, as did Rosie in the bed next to mine. I think they were feeling sorry for me still having to wait for my op.

Amanda came over with a form and asked me more of the same questions I had been asked since the whole thing had begun.

The TV above my bed was on. Apparently there was still £3.50 credit on it, so I was also able to use the phone on it as well but didn't feel like ringing anyone at that time, I just wanted to get the op over and done with.

Unfortunately, I kept seeing programmes and adverts on the TV showing food and my stomach was now rumbling!

Midday: My blood pressure was taken and a peg was put on my finger to determine oxygen and blood levels or something. My temperature was taken via the usual thermometer stuck under my tongue, which revealed a measurement of 36.7 (apparently in the middle of the norm.)

I chatted to three other patients in the ward who were awake, opposite and next to me, then my calves were measured for those glamorous, tight surgical socks – the ones with big circular holes in the soles of your feet, presumably to allow them to "breathe" due to the tight squeezing around the rest of the leg! My right calf was apparently slightly bigger than my left, which surprised me but not the nurse measuring me. She said that was quite normal. Oh good.

Simon eventually returned and I suggested he might as well go home now, especially as staying would have meant feeding the car park meter again, which had expired at 12.30. There was no telling how long it would be before my operation. He agreed and dutifully went, saying he would come back later.

12.30: I was still waiting. I played with the bed buttons (don't tell the nurses!). I rose the back of the bed up by the many pillows, then down, then up again! OK so I'm a big kid!

Lunchtime came, then tea, coffee and biscuits, but not for me. Well, I wanted to go on a diet anyway!

I was passed a menu for the next day's meals for me to book but reading through this only succeeded in making me even hungrier! Still, at least I knew what would be coming to me the next day.

1.40: I sat on the edge of the bed, switched the light on and off with the remote control (don't tell the nurses that, either!) Amanda, wheeling a trolley into the ward, saw me and laughed (don't tell her supervisor!). I justified it with "I'm bored!"

The other patients couldn't believe I was still waiting and you could sense the sympathy in their voices when we spoke. Rosie voiced her disbelief and concern inbetween reading her book. Caroline, in the bed diagonally opposite mine, occasionally sympathised whilst doing Sodoku.

2 pm: I asked the male nurse, Andy, how much longer he thought I might have to wait. He found out that there were two other patients in front of me, so I asked if there was anything I could do for them (the nurses, not the patients!). I said I could write my name on the board above my bed, because mine was the only board with nothing written on it (apart from C4!). He said yes and could I also write DJF (my surgeon's initials) and NBM. "Nil by mouth?" I asked. He nodded.

He gave me a black marker pen to do the job. I wrote everything on the large, beige coloured board and, underneath the initials NBM, I wrote '(hungry)'. Amanda saw this and commented: "It won't work!"

I wandered back to the nurses' station to return the marker. No-one was there. I was about the place it in the box on the desk with the other pens when I noticed the large white board attached to the opposite ward (the one I was in last year). On it was written the name of all the patients and allocated bed numbers. I noticed my name was spelt incorrectly, as it usually is. I couldn't resist amending it, as well as changing the "Ms" to "Mrs". Well, what's that saying about the devil finding work for idle hands....? (Gosh - I hope none of the staff ever reads this!)

A little while later I returned to the nurses' station, stating I was thirsty and, if I couldn't have a drink of water, could I perhaps have a polo mint instead? Andy sympathised but explained that, if I was to do this and suddenly there was an "opening" in the schedule for me, I would then have to wait at least another two hours before they could operate on me, so was it really worth it? I reluctantly agreed to remain thirsty and keep my fingers crossed.

4 pm (approx.) An anaesthetist came and introduced himself and we went through any allergies I may have – the only one, I told him, if you could call it that, was "general anaesthetic"! I explained how I was prone to vomiting immediately after an operation and that, once, I vomited

so much I burst my stitches and had to be rushed back into surgery, this time using a local anaesthetic. I remember wearing an oxygen mask and I could actually feel all the stitches entering my body...and it was a particularly personal part of the body too! I mentioned that the lumpectomy op last year didn't produce such feelings, though, and he said he would probably use the same anaesthetics then.

Shortly afterwards I was advised to put on my hospital gown and prepare to go to theatre. Wow! At last! What a way to make you get excited about an operation – just delay it a long time!

Nurse Sandie came to put my *tight* socks on once I had finally been given the OK to prepare for my op. Unfortunately, these were so tight, she struggled to get the first one over my foot before I was grimacing in pain, telling her to take it off! Although they had to be fairly tight, even she thought these ones were much too tight for the job so she went and replaced them with a slightly more comfortable pair.

She was a similar age to myself, probably younger, with short, blonde wavy 'Marilyn Monroe'-style hair. She had my kind of sense of humour and we got on well. I told her about the time I was being wheeled to theatre many years ago at Frimley, Surrey, which coincided with a particular ad on the TV illustrating someone being wheeled to theatre, when the patient sat up and sang. I couldn't resist sitting up from the trolley myself and singing the same line from the Nat King Cole song (used in the ad) "There may be trouble ahead....". She laughed and had one or two suggestions of her own for me to sing this time, including the Peter Cook/Dudley Moore tune "Goodbyeee...goodbyeee....Wipe a tear, baby dear, from your eyeee!" She suggested I wave to my boob at the same time!

I went to the nurses' station and asked when I would actually be "going in", only I was getting cold wearing just a gown! One of the nurses there was apparently a theatre nurse and replied "Now"!

I was shocked.

"*Right* now?" I asked.

"Yes," came the curt reply.

"Have you changed your mind?" Andy smiled.

"No! No!" I replied, "Only, I'll just go and tell the other patients – am I walking to theatre?"

They said that I was, so I dashed back to the ward and exclaimed with delight that my time had come! They were pleased for me! (Probably more pleased to get rid of me!)

I had to walk to the theatre, carrying a pillow, accompanied by the theatre nurse. I was getting used to the procedure.

When I arrived in the ante-room I was told to lie on the theatre bed whilst they did the usual OBS. There was a lot of medical equipment all around. Mr Ferguson was there – as usual unrecognisable in his cap and gown. He examined my breast and looked closely at it. I couldn't resist it and quipped: "Are you going to put 'R.I.P.' on it?!" I sort of got a response from those around me. I don't think medical staff are used to patients like me......

Anyway, he and one of the nurses began having a little difficulty inserting a canula into the back of my hand and had to withdraw it (the canula, not my hand), making a second attempt in a different vein. The nurse held my wrist fairly tight, as instructed by Mr Ferguson, whilst he was holding my hand, trying to insert the canula again. I was naturally looking in the other direction and I remember thinking what soft hands he had! When I mentioned this to Simon some days later, he replied "Well, I should think so! You wouldn't want to be operated on by someone with hands like mine, would you?" Simon has large, masculine hands, befitting someone in his construction trade!

They eventually, between them, managed to insert the canula successfully, then Mr Ferguson went to the double doors ahead of me and, as he opened one, he gave a broad smile and called over to me; "Bye! You'll be fine, don't worry!" I must have needed reassuring, as this actually reassured me!

I don't remember much after that. With previous operations, I was told by the anaesthetist to just start counting to ten and I never got past five! However, on this occasion I didn't even realise I had been given the anaesthetic before I must have "fallen asleep"!

The next thing I knew, I was slowly waking on a bed in a large "recovery" room. A nurse was beside me. There were many other beds in the room and lots of equipment. I remembered seeing a lot of "white" everywhere – the walls, ceiling, furniture - which I saw through my hazy eyes! After a little while (which was apparently an hour but seemed like two minutes!), they wheeled me back to my ward. At least I didn't have to walk this time – I couldn't even sit up!

CHAPTER TWENTY-NINE

Jan is Busting Out All Over!

Simon came and visited me that evening. Naturally, I couldn't converse much but I was glad to see him. I told him it was just as well he went home when he did as I didn't have my op until after 4 pm!

Around 10 am, the morning after the op, I was a little weak on my legs. A nurse walked with me to the bathroom so I could use the toilet. She then returned with me to my bed so that I could gather my toiletries and accompanied me to the bathroom again. I had a "wound drain" attached to my chest area, similar to the one I had had after my lumpectomy op last year. There were a few mls of blood collecting in the bulbous area leading to the white plastic bag. I was told that I should not get as much of a discharge this time, though, as it was the removal of the lymph gland nodes that caused excessive fluids to be released before.

Once in the bathroom, the nurse asked if I wanted to see my wound whilst there was someone with me. I walked up to the wall mirror and stared at my reflection, dressed in a blue hospital gown. I was a little apprehensive at first, casting my mind back to visions of the photographs Annie had shown me. Then I boldly announced "Well, it's there whether I look or not!".

I removed my gown and gazed at my chest for a while. One "full" breast, as Mr Ferguson has called it, dangling next to...well....nothing really. There was no bruising, just a lot of dressing and tape. All you could see of my semi-flat chest area through the taping was a thin, slightly jagged, dark, horizontal line where once rose a "full", if deformed (from lumpectomy) breast!

It wasn't as bad as I thought it would be, and I told the nurse so. She asked if I wanted the door left ajar when washing, to which I replied "Not likely!". She left me to get washed in the sink under the other mirror which was nearest to the door. I laid my gown over a rail, leaving me semi-naked, wearing only a pair of briefs. I proceeded to wash my face then dry it with my towel. Suddenly, I could feel my whole face and head getting very hot; I knew I'd had this before, when I was in that café last year – and just before I collapsed. I knew I had to get someone back in – fast. I saw a red cord dangling nearby and pulled it.

The next thing I knew I was lying on the floor in a foetal position, with my face next to a large, round door stop. I was topless but was clear-headed enough to think thank Heavens I had my knickers on! I could hear voices outside. I felt like I was dreaming and was so, unbelievably, tired. I didn't want to, and indeed couldn't, move at all. The people on the other side of the door seemed to be having trouble getting in – probably because my legs were blocking the door. I kept feeling a slight "push" of the door against my bottom, as I was facing away from the door.

"Try the other side!" one of them said.

They eventually burst in – hoards of people in nurses' uniforms. One of them kneeled on the floor next to me and asked if I knew what I had fallen on. Apparently I had hit my nose and had a red mark across the bridge! I slowly looked around, unable to raise my head very much. I assumed it was the large door stop that had caused it but it could equally have been the sink, I didn't really know. She commented that she thought I couldn't have finished that quickly when she heard the bell – she had only left me for a few minutes!

I felt them trying to lift me up. One of them tried to put my gown back on me in an effort to make me look decent. She had a bit of a struggle on her hands, as I was like a floppy doll!

They managed, between them, to lift me onto a chair and I must have fainted again. When I came to I looked down in front of my gown and could see bits of vomit trailing down it.

Now I wouldn't really consider myself particularly fat or heavy (although, since chemo, I have put on a bit of weight), but these four female nurses had to enlist the help of two male porters to wheel me to my bed back at the end of the ward and attempt to lie me down!

They closed the curtains around me and put an oxygen mask on me. They did an ECG, blood est, checked the oxygen levels in my blood (through the peg on the finger thing) and struggled to remove those awful tight socks! I observed it all through what felt like a drunken haze.

A doctor in green scrubs came through the curtains. He explained that he was actually someone else's doctor. The staff nurse told him I had fainted twice and that my body had 'twitched' and my eyes rolled. I was shocked to hear all that! My eyes have never 'rolled' before! I thought I had just fainted normally! He asked me if I knew where I was. I did and told him so! He explained that he didn't think I had had a fit due to my answers – it was just a faint. So I was right – I had just fainted normally! I'd never had a fit in my life!

Shortly after he and most of the others went away, I started to feel a little sick again. I mentioned this to the one remaining nurse, who told me to turn on my side as she held one of those grey "vomit trays" under my mouth and, yes, a trail of vomit exited my mouth, like I hadn't done that enough during chemo! Oh well, at least I was used to it!

They left the oxygen mask on me for a couple of hours. I actually started to feel better because of it. However, I sat up and removed it in order to have lunch – nothing was going to stop me eating this time!

My own doctor came to see me later and confirmed the other doctor's notes that I had not had a fit, I was quite lucid, but my nose was still quite red – she said it would probably be bruised. Oh great! First I chipped a tooth from fainting at the café, now I would have a bruised, bumpy nose from collapsing in a bathroom! Was everything all designed to take my mind of cancer and losing a breast, I wondered?

Later, I felt better. I had struggled a bit with the shepherd's pie lunch but really enjoyed the evening meal.

The staff nurse told me I wasn't allowed out of bed the next day – apparently she had already had two patients collapse on her that day! I later discovered that other patients who had had operations were now being told to "bed rest" for two days after their operations – so my incident served some purpose then!

The young, friendly Russian patient in the bed opposite me had been waiting nearly all afternoon for the taxi to take her home. We chatted occasionally before the car finally arrived and bade each other farewell. Her replacement was a slim 77-year-old lady called Marie, who came from a town 60 miles from Dublin. I felt sorry for her – she was always in a lot of pain with her thumb, which was held up by traction. However, it didn't stop her conversing with me frequently. In fact, during one of her more pain-free periods while we were both having a cup of tea, she remarked that she liked my "masculine" haircut, thinking I had deliberately styled it that way! I thought I looked like a skinhead, mature tomboy but she seemed to like the "salt and pepper" stubbled head and even wanted the same style herself! I felt obliged to inform her it was due to my cancer treatment and she immediately sympathised.

1/2/09: I was wheeled, on a chair, to a different bathroom to use the toilet. (I wasn't keen on returning to the other bathroom – bad memories and all that!) On arrival, I rose from the chair, which was left outside, and the accompanying nurse told me to ring to let her know when I was ready to be wheeled back.

Inside the bathroom, once ready to leave, I couldn't locate a cord to pull. I was loathe to stand for too long after what had happened before. I spotted a red button on the wall with faint, black lettering: "E M E......G...NY". In my hurry not to be kept waiting, I pushed it. Immediately, a loud, fast sounding bell rang out through all the wards.

I walked out of the bathroom, noticed the chair still outside, then my eyes fell upon two female nurses rushing towards me from the nurses' station like Batman and Robin! I called to them, apologetically, that it wasn't an emergency – realising what the faint word on the button was meant to read!

The hospital Pharmacist, a Spanish lady, did her rounds, asking everyone what painkillers they liked (I mean, needed to take) and when she came to me I told her I wasn't in pain – except when I bashed my nose after falling in the bathroom! She said she liked people like me – who don't need painkillers – makes her job easier!

Caroline had been discharged today and was all packed and ready for her husband to come and take her home. However, when he eventually got back to her on the phone, he said he would meet her in the main reception of the hospital – which was very, very far away from our ward. I felt sorry for her. She was clearly in a lot of physical pain (somewhere around her stomach). She, like me, had a wound drain attached, which you could see below her clothes. However, for whatever reason (perhaps he felt guilty), he did eventually come up to the ward in the end to take her home.

I had given mum the telephone number of the phone attached to the modern TV screen (on which one also had access to the internet – I ask you; who feels like 'surfing the net' after an operation?). Unfortunately, the one time we spoke on the phone was cut short due to the expiry of the money which had been put in by the previous patient. That meant no TV for me either! When I had paid for Nick to have use of the TV a couple of years previously when he had a minor op. they said unused funds would be refunded. He was discharged early and we never got the money back (quite a tidy sum, too). Hence I was loathe to feed such a machine again, preferring instead to do without and just annoy the other patients and their families by chattering to them a lot! (I don't *think* they minded but I did notice their "goodbyes" when I left were quite ecstatic!)

The petite, lively 95-year-old Katharine in the bed in the far corner had waited a while to have her op but the next day she was more or less back to her normal, pleasant self. Her son Peter visited fairly regularly – he even helped me sort out a phone query I had – I was curious to know if I could still receive incoming calls if the TV screen was off (which it now was), so he kindly rang the phone number to find out. My phone rang, so my question was answered.

Simon and Nick visited me that day. I was wary of Nick trying to play with my mattress again, like he did in the other ward! And yes, he couldn't resist, even when I was on it!

Apparently, most of Britain had had the worst snow in twenty years today, except the South West, which was good news for us in Devon!

2/2/09: Started snowing in Devon today! However, it wasn't as bad as the south east of England. It had completely thawed and vanished by the evening due to warm sunshine!

During the day our ward was visited by half a dozen suited, middle-aged gentleman who were examining everything in sight (except us patients!). They peered into all the nooks and crannies and one of them even ran his finger along the top of my bed curtain rails (he must have been quite tall!) and eventually they began revealing who they were by the questions they were asking us – hospital inspectors! They asked us if we found the temperature was alright and one of them asked if it was OK for me, being right next to the window, did the radiator work properly, etc.? I replied yes, although I had noticed a slight breeze blowing the curtain at night, even though the window was double-glazed, but otherwise it was OK. I had plenty of blankets on me.

Another of them threw open a question about how we found the food. I resisted the urge to say we didn't find it, it was given to us on a tray, and instead gave my two-penny-worth opinion, that I actually found it quite good and tasty – although larger portions wouldn't have gone amiss! He seemed pleased with my opinion about the quality, but not so much the quantity issue. He nonchalantly followed the others as they strolled out of the ward, no doubt to scribble down their findings before pouncing onto the next unsuspecting department!

I was amazed to be told by a doctor that I could go home today if I felt OK (I was actually paying visits to the bathroom unaccompanied now!). So I rang Simon to pick me up if he could. A nurse came round to my bed to tell me they had contacted a Breast Care Nurse to come and see me soon. However, it was just my luck that she discussed my very personal situation only a foot away from a male electrician who was bending down next to wall sockets near my bed (doing safety checks or something – on the sockets, not my bed)!

She advised me that, if my drain was still draining in seven days' time, I should notify the hospital (presumably so something could be done about it, not to boast about it!)

A little while later, Sandra, one of the Breast Care Nurses, arrived to see me.

"I hear you've had a bit of excitement during your stay here," was her opening greeting.

I briefly related the details of my "fainting" episode, saying it seems to be a habit of mine, having also done the same at a café last year!

"Still, the book was getting boring," I said, "At least these events give me something different to write about instead of 'had chemo, vomited, had chemo, vomited'!"

She asked to see my selection of bras to see if any would be suitable to wear with a "cumfie".

She sifted through my collection.

"No....not this one...no..." she mumbled whilst discarding each of my fourteen (some new), mostly under-wired bras. Finally, she thought one of my sports bras would be the most ideal for now, until I could buy a proper "mastectomy" bra. She had a couple of cumfies for me to wear, which I was pleased about. She suggested I inserted them into the bra now, using miniscule safety pins she provided, and get dressed.

I put on my favourite, bright red polo neck jumper. I must have been in quite a good mood (or silly mood) because I remember pointing to the red blood in the drain and announcing, quite cheerfully, "Look – it matches my jumper!" I was probably just pleased it was all over and I would soon be on my way back home.

"Do you want to come and see yourself in the mirror?" she asked. Of course I did, so we went to *that* bathroom, where I rushed to face the mirror which revealed your reflection to waist level. I was thrilled to see a full, complete, convincing chest again and beamed: "I'm a woman again!"

Upon discharge I was given a leaflet regarding the drain that was attached to me.

I was concerned that I might need to make frequent visits back to the hospital for fluid drainage from my body, as before. However, Sandra reassured me that the reason it was so frequent last time was due to the lymph glands, which produce the body fluid. As there were no lymph glands involved this time, the problem shouldn't be half as bad. She confirmed that it should be removed once the fluid content in the drainage bag had reduced to 50mls or lower, adding that Mr Ferguson usually liked them removed after seven days anyway. As before, a District Nurse would visit me every day to check on this and do whatever was necessary (like listen to my poor jokes).

Within half an hour of me ringing him, Simon surprised me by turning up ready to collect me. He obtained a wheelchair (I think it was mostly from seeing how much luggage I had – mostly bras!) We left at 1.30, saying goodbye to patients and staff alike, as he whizzed me to the lift and onwards home!

CHAPTER THIRTY

There's Something I've Got to Get Off My Chest....

Once I got home I remembered to read from the literature the hospital had sent me prior to admission, including what to do when leaving! Somewhat late now, I know! Still, I felt fairly au fait with procedures now anyway, fortunately.

3/2/09: I weighed myself today. I actually lost a little weight! (only a few pounds, but that was enough to cheer me up.) Then it dawned on me – of course....it was interesting to realise that that was exactly how much my boob must have weighed. I had no idea they were so heavy – you don't notice when they're attached to you (well, unless you're *really* big, I suppose).

I related to the District Nurse, my "fainting" episode at the hospital. She laughed and said only *I* would do something like that! She checked the wound and drainage bag. I was dismayed to see the blood level in it had gone *up* to 100ml so she replaced the bag.

Nick had a two hour driving lesson in Exeter.

4/2/09: The next day, another District Nurse drained my blood (they all sound like vampires!) and I was relieved to see the amount in the bag had now gone down to a more respectable 40ml.

Later in the day, I noticed something peculiar about my chest – and I'm not referring to the absence of a breast! Between the scar and my remaining boob, there appeared to be a little "bump" (about an inch in length and centimetre depth) underneath the dressing tape. There was a pea-sized blob of dried blood right in the middle of the bump, prompting Simon to comment: "It looks like an eye!" He was prone to remarks like that, you might have gathered. He also took great delight in teasing me about another sore point – my hair – calling me Tintin, due to the slight quiff that was growing. Well at least it *was* growing....slowly but surely...albeit in strange directions!

That evening I was itching like mad at the insertion point of the drain, also having pressure from the part of my bra which was touching it. I hoped the nurse would be able to remove the drain the next day.

5/2/09: Drain was removed. Hooray!

Snow came back to the South West with a vengeance and with no sun around there was very little thawing, if any. I was just glad I wasn't out there driving a car.

Gina rang to see how I was doing, post-op, which was kind of her. So I told her.

My brother in law Chris and his fiancée Susan (they recently announced their engagement!) were always in touch by phone or email, as were many other friends and relations, which was really nice and thoughtful.

Local elections were brewing. I rang the Conservative councillor to get his views on local entertainment facilities (I was thinking of my drama group). We had a long chat, at the end of which he wanted to know which way I was voting. I didn't know myself until I had spoken to all of the councillors and told him so!

6/2/09: Sandra (Breast Care Nurse) rang to check on me (probably worried about my comparing body fluid colours to clothing!)

The District Nurse checked on my wound site. Seemed OK.

7/2/09: I was slowly growing another boob due to the fluid disbursement – Yay! (OK, I knew it wasn't going to last.) I eventually became brave and removed the plaster and dressing from the site. I was impressed with how it looked – less bloody too!

Lying in bed I contemplated the clever design of our bodies; everything is duplicated but anything that isn't and is solitary (i.e. nose, mouth), is placed *centrally* so as not to make you lop-sided – like I was now. I almost felt like my remaining breast was awkward and in the way. (Not that I advocated removal...no...not if it wasn't absolutely necessary). But I definitely felt more "balanced" when wearing my cumfie in a bra. We women were meant to have either two breasts or none (preferably the former).

Alix returned my call. I mentioned about the Amazonian warrior women cutting off their own breasts to facilitate using bows and arrows, to which she replied I was like them – "I said you were a fighter!" she said.

"But I would need my *right* breast removed if I wanted to use a bow and arrow, not my left one!" I replied.

She said she wanted a copy of my book to read. OK Alix. This is it!

In bed that night I found myself constantly taking deep breaths in bed. I found it very hard to breathe. Was this some kind of panic attack? I don't know. I didn't know how I was going to get to sleep. Still, I was relieved that I did eventually. I knew I must have done because the next morning I woke up!

It rained today. (Got to keep up with the weather reports!)

My cousin Sharyl and dad and brother rang to speak to me (not all at the same time!). I related to Steve all the incidents that had happened, including my second "collapse" at the hospital. He remarked that I was very "matter of fact" about it all, especially regarding the pain I had suffered. He thought, perhaps, I should be in the SAS because nothing seemed to bother me! (Little did he know – about pain, not the SAS!). Or else I should consider becoming a boxer (making reference to my chipped tooth and bashed nose from both occasions!) Either that or, he suggested, I should always wear gum shields or something covering my face, in case it ever happened again! Hmm...

Sometimes it felt like my right breast was too big and heavy for my body now that it was "on its own". Still, I reconciled myself to the fact that it was probably just something I would have to get used.

9/2/09: Christine visited at midday with a "Get Well" card and lots of their own, farm-grown apples! She stayed for a while and we chatted over a cup of tea (one each, that is!)

Observing the slow but ever changing growth of hair on my head, Simon remarked that I now had a "GI Jane" hairstyle!

Today it felt like I was finally beginning to "see the light at the end of the tunnel". It was the best I had felt about myself for ages. A peculiar thing happened as I was writing that note for this book – the "long life" lightbulb dangling from our bedroom ceiling suddenly brightened! Freaky or what?

Unfortunately, I was now beginning to experience what I believe is known as "prickly heat", generally during my increasingly frequent "hot flushes". I just had to put up with it – it never lasted very long – no more than a minute or so, I'd say.

10/2/09:   I felt a twinge in my stomach whilst perusing the internet. Nothing very significant about that, you might say, and you'd be right. But not a lot else happened that day! Well, apart from Nick having an interview at the local, large garden centre at 11 am.

I also received a lovely bunch of flowers from Heather, Gary and the boys. Later that day the local Lib-Dem councillor, who lives nearby, came round as I wanted her opinion regarding local entertainment facilities. We also discussed my probable inability to vote in person due to my condition so she advised a postal vote.

Bedtime: Simon and I were discussing the various nicknames he had been giving me, due mostly to my hair (well, that's what some people do when they go to bed...discuss nicknames!) We recalled the various ones like Tufty, GI Jane, Tin Tin, then just as he said the last one, he happened to notice the cartoon image on my blue nightie – it was a cute white terrier, with the words "Scruffy Pup" emblazoned beneath it. As usual, Simon couldn't resist: "Oh look!" he pointed to the picture of the dog, "There's Snowy!" For those too young to understand the significance, that was Tin Tin's dog and my "Scruffy Pup" looked just like him! Needless to say I fell asleep soon after that!

CHAPTER THIRTY-ONE

Smile Please!

11/2/09: The day had come when I would, hopefully, find out more about my cancer, i.e. if removing my breast had removed the cancer, or if the cancer cells had just been sneaky and escaped elsewhere, like they did when they set up camp under my arm with the lymph nodes.

I was being picked up by Mary (Hospiscare) to travel to the hospital for my "follow up" appointment with the surgeon.

I tried to mentally prepare myself for whatever I was going to be told because, after all, there was nothing I could do about it, other than what they told me. Anyway, I considered there wasn't much else they *could* do for me – except to say that the cancer had spread.....

I decided not to wear my wig as my hair was (very slowly) beginning to look respectable, albeit somewhat masculine.

It was 2.15 when I spotted her new hatchback car pull up outside our drive. I quickly grabbed my long, grey ('Darth Vader') cardigan and threw it on, rushing to the front door in order to save her getting out of her car. I opened the door and jumped backwards in shock because she was already standing on the steps immediately on the other side, her finger poised at our doorbell. She too, was obviously surprised at seeing the door open before she had had a chance to ring the bell. It was hard to tell who had the biggest fright and this led us both into hysterics, all the way to her car!

During the journey she mentioned how busy she had been yesterday due to lots of patients being ferried to and fro, who should have been seen the previous Friday, but couldn't due to the heavy snow we had experienced. She mentioned how yesterday was the busiest day for traffic she had ever known and made reference to the fact that she had been driving for ten years now and I couldn't help but interrupt her with "Aren't your arms tired?". She burst into laughter and replied "No, but my bottom is!"

She asked if I needed her to come with me to the appointment but I said I would be OK and that these "follow up" appointments usually take quite a while due to the waiting time anyway. So she gave me her mobile phone number just in case I finished early and went on her way to another appointment.

Once inside, I discovered the lift was out of action so I walked up the one flight of steps leading to Surgical Outpatients.

At reception, one of the nurses overheard my request and began laughing. Instead of my asking the Receptionist how long I would have to wait for my appointment (even though I was on time), I actually phrased it "How far is he behind schedule today?!" She said she would find out for me.

The large waiting area was quite busy. I found a seat near the "walkways" which ran the perimeter of the area surrounding the rows of seats and sat near a friendly and chatty "mature" couple who were also waiting to be seen.

Shortly after I settled into my seat, a nurse came up to me and very apologetically announced that the wait would be about half an hour. I replied that that was better than the usual two hours, so I didn't mind at all.

The couple near me obviously overhead this and we began discussing waiting times generally, before going onto more serious subjects, like the appearance of the doctors! I said I was under Mr Ferguson and added how I always found that to be a strange expression. The wife and I ended up in laughter, and she told her husband (the patient, apparently) that he wasn't going to be seeing the 'good-looking one'! I doubt if that upset him because we were referring to the male of the species. Although....you never know.....

Her husband was cheery, around 60/65 and quite tall. How did I know that if he was sitting down, I hear you ask. Well they had to stand up when they were called to see his doctor and I could see he was very tall! He had a fluorescent blue walking stick – I said I'd like a car that colour! His wife said he had fallen down a flight of stairs at the hospital. I said I couldn't beat that – I had only fainted in a hospital bathroom!

I took out my little notebook and began making notes for this book. I felt a little self-conscious and piped up "I must look like a reporter!" They both smiled.

They were eventually called in before me at 3.10 (I noted the time because I had nothing else to do except write notes). Soon after they exited the consulting room, caught my eye and waved a cheery goodbye.

A nurse caught my attention and passed on a message to me from Mary; something about the time she would be able to come and pick me up, so there was no need for me to ring her. I thanked her, then noticed one of the large, glossy magazines on the coffee table – the one that's all photos of celebrities (mostly weddings,, etc.), you know the one I mean – the one that sounds like a greeting! Anyway, I happened to notice it advertising an article inside about Kylie Minogue who, of course, also had breast cancer. I put my notebook away and picked up the magazine, passing the remaining waiting time by reading said article, which was quite interesting as it turned out.

Finally, it was my turn to be seen. A nurse showed me into a little room next to an office, complete with trolley bed, chairs, sink, pile of gowns, surgical gloves – the usual medical paraphernalia. She gave me a "half gown", much like the one I had to wear for the mammogram, and told me to change into it. She then left and I did as instructed. I sat on the edge of the bed, my feet dangling like a little girl, periodically checking my gown was done up properly, though why I bothered I have no idea – I would be exposing myself shortly when the surgeon came in anyway!

I found myself reading signs on the walls, like the big poster that said something like "A patients acquires an infection every two hours...." and instructing staff to always wash their hands. I thought I wouldn't like to be that patient, getting an infection every two hours! At least there were a lot of these notices around the hospital. It was quite a clean place really, fortunately!

I started to get a little cold – those gowns are quite loose and not very warm! After 20 minutes the connecting door opened and in walked Breast Care Nurse Annie and Mr Ferguson. They asked how I was and Mr Ferguson asked to see the scar. He was obviously impressed with his own work! He said the scar was very good, the wound was healing well. He could tell it needed draining as it seemed like I was slowly growing another boob! So he went ahead and drained the fluid from my body using a large syringe needle whilst Annie held the tray to catch the fluid, which was reddish-orange in colour. Whilst they carried out the procedure, I remarked that they would soon be burning me (radiotherapy) and were now stabbing me! They laughed and said they prefer to give the treatment different names!

I mentioned that sometimes it felt like I still had a breast when I occasionally get an itch, so I can now understand how people feel who have limbs amputated but feel as though they have still got them.

Once he had finished draining me, Mr Ferguson asked if I would mind having my photo taken of the scar area with a digital camera. It was obviously to be added to the folder of other photos I had been shown before the op. (I hope!) I said that seeing such photos definitely helped me, so I agreed. He nipped back into his office. I turned to Annie and said "Oh no, I've hardly got any make up on!" She laughed and explained he wouldn't be taking one with my face in it! I was relieved.

He reappeared holding his digi-camera and got me to stand in front of him. There was no point in smiling for the camera, I just commented "There aren't many men I'd allow to take a photo of me semi-naked!"

He snapped once or twice, put the camera away and said "And now I suppose you want to know the results..."

I thought he was going to show me the picture in the camera then realised he was referring to my cancer. "Oh yes, definitely," I replied.

He told me they had analysed the breast tissue that had been removed during my operation and discovered that I was "clear" with no trace of cancer! That was great news!

"Do I still have to go through radiotherapy then?" I asked.

Unfortunately, his answer was yes – it was their kind of 'belt and braces' approach. Annie added that it wouldn't be for at least six weeks though. I was pleased – mainly because I had lots of drama group appointments, meetings, etc. to attend. She was obviously surprised. She said most patients to whom she had given this news were quite upset at the delay, but not me! (I wasn't looking forward to it anyway.) Referring to tiredness, Mr Ferguson said that I wouldn't be back to normal until six weeks after radiotherapy. He added that he wouldn't see me for six months, smiled broadly and shook my hand. I thanked him for his help and he returned to his office, ready to print the photo of my chest!

I got dressed then Annie and I sat on the edge of the bed so she could go through a few things with me.

Before she began I asked her excitedly:

"What did he say?"

She smiled and replied;

"You're 'all clear'. There's no trace of cancer cells in that area now."

She asked if I understood everything Mr Ferguson had said and what had happened. I thought I had. I just wanted confirmation! She said that I would now be put on the 'mammogram register' when I was 55 until I was 74. We both thought that was an odd age for it to stop. Why not 75? Or 74 and three quarters?! I would also be seen six monthly by the hospital for two years for a check up, then annually for three years after that.

She commented that no-one would ever tell me I was 'cured'. I realised later that this was because there was always the possibility the cancer could return, e.g. 'secondary cancer' etc. So obviously there was no cure as such yet.

We discussed prosthetic boobs. I told her that the one I had held at a previous meeting seemed quite heavy, but she reassured me that the main prosthetic boob (not the cumfie) could be lighter than the one I held then.

When we said goodbye, I walked slowly through the waiting area, past many patients. I wanted to grin broadly, even laugh, but I thought about how some of them might not have had good news like me and it wouldn't be very tactful of me to boast about my present good fortune in such a way. However, I couldn't keep it bottled up forever. As I passed the reception desk, I was pleased to see there was at least one person there – the nurse who had passed Mary's message on to me earlier. Good. I'll tell her, I thought. As I breezed past the desk I called out (but not too loudly) "I'm cancer free!" I was surprised at how pleased she was for me. We didn't know each other at all. She actually came around the desk and gave me a hug. I felt great! She was a lot smaller than me (but I am tall) so I didn't want to squash her! As it happens, talk about a small world, it turned out that her husband was in Sales at Hospiscare and knew Mary, my driver! We chatted briefly before bidding each other farewell.

I hadn't gone more than twenty paces down the first corridor when I actually saw Mary coming towards me. At least we didn't frighten each other this time!

I couldn't stop talking in the car all the way home. I said it was like being given a new lease of life and all I wanted to do was to stand on top of one of the many hills we were passing and shout "I'm alive!"

Fortunately Mary was more than understanding and said she wouldn't blame me!

She dropped me off half an hour later. I waved goodbye to her as she drove off and I started to walk, somewhat excitedly, down the driveway path. It was no good – before I could ring anyone to give them the good news, I had to pop into our neighbour's first. Margaret insisted I enter their bungalow and gave me tea and biscuits. She hadn't seen my new "hair" before and actually said she liked it! Some people are so polite! (Simon: take note!) She seemed very relieved at my news and told me to take a seat on the sofa. Whilst drinking my tea I was particularly taken by one of the comments she made: "the NHS saved your life". I repeated the words thoughtfully...."the NHS saved my life....yes....they did..." and finished my tea.

A little while later I thanked her for the tea, saying I should really get home so I could tell everyone else – mostly Simon!

And that was just what I did – I rang everyone! (Had an expensive phone bill that month, but I no longer cared about money now!) Unfortunately, I couldn't get hold of Simon – he was busy at work, so I left a message. So I rang his mum and dad, my dad and brother, Sharyl, Simon's brothers, friends and everyone who had been in touch with me from the beginning. I was just in the middle of speaking to Jerry (drama group) when I heard pips on the phone. I felt a bit rude telling him I needed to cut short our conversation because I suspected they were from Simon, trying to get through to me, and I was right. He couldn't talk for long but at least I was able to give him the news.

That evening I suggested we celebrate the good news at our local inn. So we had a meal there at 8.30 and finished at home with a bottle of champagne we had been given at Christmas.

The next day I went on a previously planned trip to Torquay with Gill. I gave her the news also.

Life was good again (in spite of the looming radiotherapy!)

CHAPTER THIRTY-TWO

Mono-Bolly

12/2/09:   Nick passed his Driving Theory Test! The same day he was offered a job at the Garden Centre and I received a lovely bunch of flowers in a vase via Interflora from Sharyl and Uncle Bill! Things were just getting better and better!

Simon was still in a "naming" mood. To explain the latest name he had for me, I have to advise that, when my brother was a toddler (I'm sure he won't mind my mentioning what I'm about to!), he called breasts "bollies" – he obviously found that easier than saying the word "breast". I actually found that quite cute at the time. Anyway, now that I only had one breast, Simon – being aware years ago about Steve's mispronunciation and obviously still remembering it – decided it would be a hoot to now name me "Mono Bolly"!

14/2/09:   I knew the good things wouldn't last. My car began making "vibrating" noises from the steering wheel, which I had to try to find time and money to fix at some point, then my laptop broke. Oh no! Would that mean this book would never be finished? (OK – who said 'Chance would be a fine thing'?) After ringing round various computer engineers, I finally went with Nick to a computer repair shop in the same village where the café was where I had collapsed! After paying over £50 for a new lead, I decided to be brave and pop into the café and ask if they had received the flowers I had sent soon after the incident. They were surprised to see me and seemed pleased that I was OK. Apparently their customers were still asking after me – I had obviously caused quite a stir that day! I would have taken a chance and had another meal with them then, however the owner was obviously in the middle of refurbishing the place, specifically the kitchen area, so I wasn't able to do so that day. They said I was always more than welcome to dine there once he had finished it. He also said it had been very thoughtful of me (to send the flowers, not faint) but I said it was the least I could do after what I had put everyone through that day and I really appreciated everyone's help. I didn't know how else to say 'thankyou'. I said I'd give them a mention in my book so they told me their names were Lorna and Ian. So....Lorna and Ian....herewith printed official 'thanks'!

Afterwards, I took Nick to the farm, where I told Alan and Christine the news about my cancer 'all clear'. Their son, David, and Pam, one of their daughters, and her baby were also there, and they all congratulated me. Nick did a bit of driving, whilst there, for experience.

Later, Nick was telling me about one of his friends' new job at Volvo. I asked if it was 'admin' and he replied, wait for it, "No, it's full time". He clearly wasn't familiar with the word 'admin', or else misunderstood me.

Back home, I was trying to print some documents and then my printer packed up! You see – it all made up for the glorious Thursday 12th! Things were back to normal again....giving me problems!

16/2/09:   Received a nice M & S gift voucher from my dad and Steve – it was only a pity that I hadn't received it sooner, like when Gill took me to M & S near Torquay a few days ago! Still, I now had an excuse to go again!

I drove Simon to and from work today. Can't remember why. Could have been that I felt sorry for him having nowhere to park barring a mile away at the top of the very steep hill near one of the town's very old churches. He didn't mind the walk down so much as having to walk back up after a long, hard day at work and his joints were giving him gip again.

The next day Gill drove me to the Garden Centre where Nick would soon be working. She had never been before and had always wanted to go so I said I would show her the way. After buying a few items, we had a very pleasant lunch there.

That evening Simon, who had driven himself to work that day, surprised me by arriving home with a lovely bunch of six red roses! I guess he had appreciated the lift I had given him yesterday!

18/2/09: Took my car into a local garage to change the oil and air filter and do a bit of wheel balancing. That always conjures up images of a magician holding wheels up in the air balanced on sticks or something, you know the sort of thing?

Also had to raid my savings in order to purchase a new printer to replace the old one. Well, it wasn't that old but the guarantee had run out so it was easier and cheaper to buy another one than try to get it repaired.

19/2/09: Simon received a nice letter from Hospiscare, inviting him to a "Carers Meeting" at the local hospital. Unfortunately, he had to decline as were going away that weekend, staying at his parents in Berkshire. They said not to worry as he could attend the next meeting in a month's time.

Our drama group's Open Evening took place at the main church in town at 8pm. I wore my special tee-shirt with the group's logo on it, as did a few other members. Jerry kindly picked me up at 6.45 in preparation for our AGM which was held an hour before the main Open Evening, at which I would be presenting the forthcoming play with Jerry, as well as general information about the group. Unfortunately, though, no-one had told me about the change of venue and I had given information to potential newcomers about where to meet without knowing of the change. However, fortunately, our secretary had posted up notices on the doors of the wrong venue to point them in the right direction! At least one of them managed to find us anyway! Both meetings went very well, will Gill volunteering to address those in attendance to announce the news of my cancer 'all clear'. When she had finished, I told them it was just to "keep them abreast of the situation"! At the end of the meeting, several members, including Nicki, Helen and Dave, all expressed how pleased they were to hear that news.

20/2/09:   Simon, Nick and I visited his parents and also picked up a car for Nick which Mark, one of Simon's brothers, had managed to purchase for him. After dinner he, his wife Cathy and their family also visited Simon's parents, as did his brother Chris and Susan (he has many siblings!) We all sat around the lounge with cups of tea or coffee and cake and chatted about...well....everything!

Simon's dad was 92 the next day, which was celebrated by Simon's mum, dad and ourselves having a pre-arranged dinner in the evening at their neighbours and mutual friends, Brenda and Alan. We played card games after dinner followed by a "bomb" game (not as dangerous as it sounds!), which we all enjoyed (you had to think of words beginning or ending with certain chosen letters before a buzzer sounded from inside a little black ball!).

Before that, Simon and I popped round to see his old boss (not in age) from before we had moved to this area. He wasn't in but his wife was and I discovered that she, too, had had breast cancer and had got the 'all clear' seven years ago. She apparently had not experienced any vomiting (unlike me), however, due to the constant canula insertion into the back of her hand (for chemotherapy), she no longer had any veins in that hand now. I avoided that due to having the Hickman Line in me and I was now glad that I had! The doctors did warn me of such consequences if I didn't have one and I now realised they were right.

Soon after we returned to his mum and dad's house, another of his brothers, Tim, and his wife Tracey and family visited to see us and stayed for a while before we had to go next door for dinner (and the bomb!) *(I hope no-one ever reads this out of context!)*

22/2/09:   We returned home.

24/2/09:   Gill called for me 10.30 to go to Torquay. We had dinner here before going on to town for a read-through of our drama group's next play.

25/2/09:   10.30: Nick started his new job at the garden centre as

Customer Services Assistant. He was particularly thrilled to have his own 'walkie talkie' on him when he worked in the centre! (Must be a teenage thing to be excited at that!) He even got tips from helping old dears wheel their trollies and load their cars with their goods (he liked that even more – the 'tips' bit I mean!) I paused writing this book to pick him up at 5.30. (It's only abour four miles away....down narrow, winding country lanes, which I'm hopeless at negotiating...give me a motorway any time!)

26/2/09: Had yet another dream last night about my hair being longer than it is and dark <u>brown</u>! Everyone, like Simon's mum, was admiring it and I was very proud of my new mane. Then I woke up. How I didn't cry when I looked in the mirror and saw my real hair I don't know.

Still, I was cheered up by what I got in the mail today: a cheque from Macmillan Cancer Support – a grant to go towards the special clothing required now that I was minus a breast, particularly mastectomy bras. I was very grateful – those things are more expensive than normal bras and my savings were now virtually depleted!

Dropped Nick off at work and went on to my 'Radiotherapy Planning' appointment at the hospital at 10 am. I waited in the 'first' waiting room before being called into the next waiting room, through double doors. The nurse handed me a nice, waist length, red and white gown with poppers on the shoulders as well as the usual place down the front. She said I could keep this for the duration as I would be needing it on a daily basis. I could just wash it as and when needed and return it at the end of the whole treatment. She pointed to some cubicles a few feet away near the large reception desk and told me to get changed and return to one of the seats near the double doors.

I entered the nearest one because the curtain was open so I knew it was vacant. There was a chair in the corner and on the left were some hooks on the wall, dangling from one of which was a very large, green plastic NHS bag for one's own clothes. To the right as you entered was a wall mirror reflecting your image to waist level. I placed my 'cancer' bag on the chair, took off my loose fitting jumper and cumfie-filled bra, put them into the green bag and examined the pretty little gown curiously. Unfortunately, it was undone and my first attempt at putting it on was a little comical, to say the least! I'd never had to wear anything before that had to be connected at the shoulders! It was like something from the TV show 'The Generation Game', as I watched myself in the mirror, trying to match up the right poppers with their counterparts. I eventually succeeded, gathered my belongings and returned to the small waiting area this side of the double doors.

I chose a comfortable-looking chair facing the large plasma TV screen, without noticing, at this time, what was being transmitted. There were about eight chairs altogether, arranged in the shape of the letter 'L', with only one other patient waiting to be seen, which I thought was a good sign – my wait might not be too long. There was a small table between the chairs with magazines and the current newspaper on display. My attention was slowly drawn to the TV programme being shown; Jeremy Kyle's show. Now I actually usually watch that programme; however, it was rather unfortunate, to say the least, that on this occasion the heading being displayed beneath the people discussing the topic read; "My children have to accept I'm dying" and it was evidently about a poor woman who had cancer. I turned to the other patient and remarked: "That's an appropriate programme to have on, isn't it?!" She agreed.

After a little while, Radiographer Dona collected me and took me into a room along the corridor, past the large reception desk. Once inside, I thought how it was reminiscent of the room where I had had my scan last year....it was like entering a sci-fi room all over again. There was a long bed in the centre of the room surrounded by a thick, steel, porthole shaped contraption and an equally large square steel object on the other side of it. Computer monitors adorned the walls and to the right was a sectioned-off ante-room, inside of which seemed to be monitoring equipment and other nurses, seen through the many windows. At least *they* would be safe when the radiotherapy sessions began!

There were a couple of chairs by the door and we both sat down. She introduced herself and began asking me questions (nothing new there) in order to complete a form she had. One question made me smile. She asked if I was pregnant! I laughed: "<u>Pregnant?</u>" I suppose I should have been flattered that she thought I was young enough for such a condition.

"Well, you're young," she continued, "We have to ask up to the age of 55..."

"<u>Young?</u>" I wondered how they referred to women who really *were* young if they call a 50-year-old woman young!

"Oh. Well I'm not...as far as I know," I replied, still a little stunned.

I was instructed to lie on the bed.

There was a wide pyramid-shaped plastic object near the end which she manoeuvred under my knees to make me more comfortable.

I complained that it was very cold underneath me.

A male radiographer who was now also in the room put a blanket on me.

"How will that help?" I asked, "My back's cold, not my front!"

"It will help retain your body heat," Dona replied.

She unpopped my shoulder poppers and the first few below my neck, opening the gown out to reveal my scar.

Dona explained everything she was going to do to me every step of the way – draw here and there, inject me here and there. All the while I was to remain perfectly still as far as I could and just relax. RELAX? That was a challenge in the circumstances...especially when faced with those big steel objects as they glided towards me before red beams of light 'marked the spot'!

My left arm was raised and my wrist and bicep were neatly placed into two black plastic 'holders' to keep it still (there are probably correct technical names for all these, but don't ask me what they are). She asked me to turn my head to the right. She maneouvred my waist to the 'correct' position. Apparently all this was in readiness for my first radiotherapy session, in order for them to be able to align the beams correctly, saving time on the day. I could now focus on the monitors along the top of the wall, one of which had large red numbers appearing on it at various times of the planning.

During the planning session, when I had to lie very still, I had an unbearable desire to scratch my itchy eyebrow! Don't ask why. I've never had an itchy eyebrow before in my life but, naturally, I just had to get one now when it was most inconvenient. I asked if I could scratch it and was politely refused.

The male radiographer sat at the desk with a computer on it near the door. I could see there were four squares on his computer screen, which he was monitoring during the procedure as the units around my bed gradually came closer and closer to my head and chest. It was easy to keep still there – fear –induced petrification enabled my lack of motion then!

The radiographers went into the little room a couple of times, telling me to relax again and keep perfectly still, before reappearing to take two digital photos.

Dona said everything seemed OK and she would just double check all was fine with Dr Goodman, the Oncologist, who was apparently in the little room as well (I hadn't even noticed him – probably because my head was facing the other way and I hadn't dared to move!).

She reappeared soon after to say he was OK with everything. I'm glad someone was!

Then his Registrar Linda, a young Muslim woman, came out of the office, asking me to sign a large consent form, much like I had to before I had the Hickman line inserted and before I had both operations.

"Ah, this is for me to sign to say if you accidentally kill me, I won't hold you responsible!"

She smiled, denying it of course, and pointed out the risks of the radiotherapy sessions (apart from big, steel equipment falling on your head? I thought). They included things like the usual nausea and vomiting (I was used to that – didn't like it much), more horrific, unexpected ones like lung inflammation, tiredness, soreness, etc. etc. I reluctantly signed the form. She then mentioned the medicine called Tamoxifen, asking if I had been taking it. I was taken aback. I told her that when this had been discussed with a hospital doctor prior to my Hickman line insertion, she agreed I wouldn't need to take it – something to do with my oestrogen and hormones and the trouble I had when I was pregnant (many years ago) – I suffered from hyperemesis (excessive sickness) for the whole nine months, spending more time in hospital than out of it, and losing two and half stone in weight in the process. My body obviously just can't handle having 'foreign matter' in it!

The Registrar asked if I could remember the doctor's name but I had seen so many in the past year, I couldn't. I probably should have made a note of it but didn't. She said she would have a word with Dr Goodman about it (the Tamoxifen, not the doctor's name).

I was told to get dressed and wait outside in the little waiting area until another nurse came to see me with information about what to expect from the treatment. Getting burnt, for a start, I imagined.

After waiting a few minutes, the Registrar appeared and told me Dr Goodman thought I should take the medicine and she arranged for me to have a prescription for the same.

Then another nurse came and took me to another little room along the same corridor. I reluctantly stuffed the prescription sheet into my bag and followed her.

It was a small room with just one empty table and a couple of chairs in it. We both sat down and she proceeded to give me the low down on what to expect. So...I could expect to be sore with redness around the area, fatigued and possibly nauseous. There was a likelihood of inflammation around the site and all side effects could last well into four to six weeks after the end of the treatment. She gave me a little leaflet with information regarding how to look after myself for the duration, including what I could and couldn't use on my skin around that area, for example, no soaps or gels with perfume, no deodorants and no sun-bathing (like that was a possibility with the rainy weather we had been having recently!). She also supplied me with a large tube of aqueous cream which I should apply to the area to help combat soreness. I told her I had just bought E45 cream, as recommended by a breast care nurse after my operation, in order to speed up the scar healing process and encourage a smoother line in that area. However, she told me that would be no good for radiotherapy treatment. I had to use the cream she had just given me.

She gave me a piece of paper showing the timetable of treatments. The first one was 9th March. I was disappointed. I told her that was the day of our 18th wedding anniversary and couldn't they re-schedule it? She said that would be near-impossible due to the machines being set for certain dates. I reluctantly agreed to the date. Not much was going my way today. Regardless, I thanked her, took the cream and went on my way.

As I drove home I recalled the words of our friend Kathy, who had also undergone radiotherapy some years previously; "you'll find radiotherapy a 'doddle' after chemotherapy!" she said. "We'll see..." I thought. My cousin Sharyl had, whilst relaying this message to a friend of hers going through the same process, inadvertently called it a "doodle"! (close!)

Back home, I became aware of more celebrities in the news with cancer. Poor Wendy Richards (of 'Eastenders' fame) had just died of cancer. What was perturbing was the fact that it was an aggressive one (like mine had been) and one which had reappeared starting in the armpit but went onto her bones and kidney.

28/2/09: Gill called round to take me to town for a bit of shopping and a cup of coffee at the local tea rooms (or was it tea at the local coffee rooms?). I mentioned that my scar was stinging and she said that was a good sign because it meant that it was healing! That sort of cheered me up.

Whilst discussing the subject, it apparently reminded her of my condition, as she commented that she had forgotten I only had one breast because I was still "bubbly and normal and, after all, was still the same person!". That cheered me up even more!

2/3/09: Nick had another two-hour driving lesson at 6pm. He had now taken to playing silly little pranks in the house, like, after coming to see me in my room to ask me something, he nonchalantly made a habit of turning on the light on our bedside cabinet, the speaker phone button and the clock radio all at the same time whenever he left! Don't ask why – I gave up long ago!

3/3/09: Snow flurries and hailstones today. Whilst with her visiting daughter, Gill had a nasty accident with her car coming down a nearby hill, due to ice on the road. She skidded and went off the road into a tree. However, if it hadn't been for the tree, it could have been a lot worse had she tumbled down the embankment. There were police cars and a fire engine there. The long 'B' road had to be closed. They were OK though, just a little shaken.

Had to take my own car into a local garage to top up my brake fluid, at a cost of £45! Yes - £45!

Caroline, our massage therapist (reminder to me: must catch up on our massages as some are still due to us!), rang to ask if it would be OK to give my telephone number to another lady who has the same condition as me. Gina had also left a message to this effect whilst I was at the garage. I said that was fine. Her name was Debbie and she lived in the same street as me. She has only lived here for a little while, originating from Great Yarmouth, just like my late Uncle Ted. Caroline gave me Debbie's number and I rang her. We arranged for her to come round to my house for a chat and a cup of tea on Thursday.

4/3/09: As expected, the weather had now turned very cold but I had to venture out into it in the evening to help run our group's auditions for the summer play (that's what happens when you're on the Casting Committee!)

5/3/09: Snowed again today!

I noticed my remaining boob was getting bigger and bigger, so my new one would have a lot of catching up to do! I couldn't stop eating! I've always been 10 ½ stone most of my adult life until recently, when it gradually crept up to 11, then 11 ½ stone after chemo. And now, suddenly, it lurched to the 12 stone mark! (Lucky I'm quite tall.) I was so dismayed...and hungry!

Toby's paw started bleeding today. I had to bathe it in salt water (couldn't find the Hibiscrub).

Later on I developed a bad migraine (not that there's such a thing as a good migraine). I started feeling nauseous and eventually was sick. I've no idea where that came from. I thought I had been on the mend. The thought of radiotherapy perhaps?

Debbie rang to apologise for not being able to come round today due to the snow, having recently had an operation on her cancer-ridden leg, she didn't want to risk falling on the snow.

During the evening, Simon and I were sitting together on the sofa, watching TV. During a break (can only converse during the commercial break!) I decided to announce my cancer news again, as if saying it aloud would mean it was true and re-affirm it.

"I've got no cancer!" I exclaimed.

"I've got no job." Simon's deadpan reply brought home to me the fact that he was shortly to join the now two-million unemployed people in this country.

6/3/09: We had a power cut today. Everything soon came back on except the TV! I had to re-set all the mains-powered equipment in the house, like clocks etc.

Spoke to Steve over the phone later. At one point we discussed pop music and Boyzone's latest single called "Better". Steve said that he heard a DJ recently introduce them thus: "And now..Boyzone are singing better!..."

I discovered today that I mustn't die my hair until a <u>year</u> after I've had chemotherapy, preferably with vegetable-based chemicals (like carrots if I want auburn coloured hair?) (Cue: depression.)

On reading the Amoena magazine, received when I purchased a mastectomy bra from them, I noticed on their letters page some letters from fellow breast cancer sufferers discussing some side-effects of the Tamoxifen drug I was meant to take. They included "damaged lungs" and bald patches on heads. Needless to say I was not a happy bunny reading that.

7/3/09: Simon and Nick picked up Nick's quadbike from Alan and Christine's farm. He didn't want to include it in their auction of items being sold off due to moving. Just meant we had to find somewhere in our tiny abode to store it now. Whilst there, they gave Alan his birthday present from us.

7.45 pm, Simon and I had a lovely three-course meal at a lavish hotel in a nearby village. It was courtesy of his parents who very kindly sent us a cheque for our anniversary, specially to have such a meal! (There was no way we could have afforded it – not now.) I wore a black glitzy cardigan and posh black skirt. I felt really cool until Simon had to comment on how the cardigan made me look like a Christmas tree! Plus, he was none too happy about the tiny pieces of glitter to be found in various places around the house, especially when they collected wherever I sat – there was no disguising where I had been because of that!

After dining, we withdrew to the large, luxurious lounge, complete with sumptuous armchairs, sofas, large fireplace, paintings, flowers and even a baby grand piano tucked away in the corner! Our coffees were brought round to us on a silver tray by the young, friendly waitress (whom Simon took a particular liking to, but we won't go into that!).

I took some photos (not of the waitresss!) and we eventually left around 11 pm, having had a thoroughly lovely time. Thank you George and Cynthia!

8/3/09: Zoe came round to visit at 1 pm and stayed for a while.

CHAPTER THIRTY-THREE

My Own Personal Heatwave!

9/3/09: Today was our 18th wedding anniversary. Today I had a slight cough and sore throat, which I believed I had caught from Simon, who had been coughing quite heavily the past day or two. Today was also the day I had to endure my first proper radiation session. Oh joy!

Ada, from Hospiscare, was my driver most of the time. On this first day she picked me up at 9 am for my 9.50 appointment at the large, modern Oncology Department. I explained that I wasn't in a position to make a donation to Hospiscare every day but that Co-ordinator Jim had agreed I could make one larger one at the very end of all my visits.

She dropped me off at the "drop off" area of the immediate car park and I ambled under a 20 yard covered walkway leading to the glass double doors. I entered the large reception area. Arrows pointed to a small tea kiosk to the left, toilets to the side of the long reception desk and another, smaller waiting area near the main Radiotherapy department through more double doors on the right.

I announced myself at reception and obtained a parking permit which would be valid for the whole three-week period I was to have my radiotherapy. It cost £3 (20p per day) and was transferable to any vehicle, which was useful! The cost was also very much cheaper than the usual car parking charges for the other car parks (which was particularly handy as I would be visiting daily). I handed this to Ada to place on her car and she bought us a cup of tea each, as there was apparently going to be a 30 minute delay before I would be seen.

We made ourselves comfortable near the outer glass wall. Ada read the local newspaper provided by the hospital and I read a magazine, but it didn't take me long to get bored. I noticed a child's miniature skittles game on the square coffee table in the middle of the room, surrounded by one section of chairs. I couldn't resist (you must know me by now!) – I just had to embarrass myself by getting up and going over to play the game (small, plastic skittles loosely attached to a 6 inch by 6 inch board, and a little plastic ball attached to a string dangling from another smaller board above them!). I unashamedly plucked the ball from its position and swung it so that it hit as many of the skittles as possible. I was quite pleased with myself, as I managed to knock down quite a few on my first attempt! It raised a few polite smiles from other patients in their chairs who didn't have anything better to do than just watch a 50 year old woman playing a child's game! God knows what Ada thought, but she didn't take me very often after that!

I gave up after a while and returned to my seat, still bored. An elderly lady sitting in the adjacent row to us, noticed the Banff tee-shirt I was wearing (from my 'wealthier' days!) and asked when I had travelled there. I explained it was a few years ago. Coincidentally, both she and Ada had also been to the same place in Canada a while back, which led to a fairly long conversation about the area before, at

10.20:   A nurse called my name and she showed me through the other double doors. She noticed I had my own gown, showing at the top of my hessian 'Cancer' bag, and instructed me to get changed in one of the nearby cubicles, as before, and to return there when ready, waiting to be called.

A few minutes later I trundled back to the small waiting area, carrying most of my clothes in a large green NHS plastic carrier bag and my own bag in my other hand, whilst draping my black, leather jacket over my arm. The TV wasn't on this time (probably just as well!). I sat on a seat nearest to the newspaper-laden coffee table and noticed the large, bold headline on the top paper. It referred to a cancer cure, so naturally I picked it up for a closer inspection. It seemed scientists thought there could possibly be a cure in about five years' time now that they were aware of a particular enzyme called 'Metastasis'. Apparently, this enzyme searches for sites in one's body in which to make 'camp' for cancer cells (sneaky little thing).

It wasn't long before my name was called and I was led by a young nurse past the long reception desk, towards a nearby narrow corridor, towards the radiotherapy theatre. The first sight that met my eyes was a square, yellow and black sign directly in front of me as I entered the corridor, before turning left. It was one of those black on yellow triangles surrounded by the words 'Caution – Radiation'. It sent subtle shivers down my spine. Now I *knew* I wasn't brave! See? I told you!

I coughed a little whilst being led down the carpeted hallway, at the end of which I had to turn into an opening on the right and into the radiotherapy room. It was quite similar, albeit smaller, to the room where I had had my radiotherapy 'planning' recently. The bed and surrounding unit were central in the room and the little room where the staff go to hide during the radiation process was to the right! (Alright, I know they're not hiding – at least, I hope not!)

I placed my belongings on the chair near the entrance and stood for a moment, gazing at the machine, the words on the sign now firmly fixed on my mind. I suppose the nurse sensed I was a little apprehensive to say the least – far more than I ever was with the chemo. I asked if it would hurt and she reassured me that I wouldn't feel a thing (why – would I be dead?). She added, though, that I may experience hot flushes later and I said that I already had them!

She introduced me to the two male nurses who were also in the room, standing either side of the bed, looking like they knew something I didn't! I recognised the tallest of them from the 'planning' day. He had dark, greying hair with glasses that did nothing to hide his good looks (there's another one I hope never reads this!) The other was a young Indian chap with a very pleasant manner whom, it later turned out, was very good at putting me at ease. He made my visits bearable.

I mentioned my slight cough and the fact that there was a possibility of my sneezing during the process. I was told this wouldn't affect anything, as long as I didn't raise my hand to my mouth whilst I was being 'radiated'! They would simply re-adjust my position on the bed. At that point I coughed again, instinctively raising my hand to cover my mouth.

"So not like that then," I said.

They told me to make myself comfortable on the bed, whilst they manoeuvred the black, plastic, triangle-shaped unit under my knees. Someone undid the poppers on my shoulder and around my left, non-existent breast. I let them get on with it and just stared above at the long, narrow gap above me in the ceiling, beside which was a notice instructing one not to look directly at it! Then they moved my 'SOS' talisman chain so that it was out of the way of the forthcoming beams. I was then told to raise my left arm and one of the nurses placed my bicep and wrist into the adjacent grips, as before.

I hadn't realised it at the time, but the room lights dimmed as I found myself the centre of attention while a lot of heads leaned over me to suss out the whereabouts of the 'tattoos' on my chest and armpit. One of them remarked that whoever had put the little black dots on me at the planning meeting must have had a very delicate hand – they were having trouble detecting them! Eventually they were found and one of the nurses drew marks on top of them (to make them stand out more, I assumed). I had to turn my head to the right, as before, and found myself staring at the wall some eight feet in the distance. Was that an 'emergency button' partially hidden from view by a couple of pillows piled on top of a lot of drawers? Should I draw their attention to it? To the right, dangling from the ceiling, was a computer monitor with lots of numbers and medical abbreviations on it.

At some point the bed I was on was raised about a foot higher.

The tall nurse grabbed me gently either side of my waist to manoeuvre my position in line with...whatever! I later learned this would inevitably happen a lot!

They asked if I was comfortable. Would *they* be? I said yes because, I suppose, under the circumstances, I wasn't too bad.

Moments later the first, circular unit was slowly and quietly manoeuvred into place about two inches from my face (though it felt like two millimetres!). I remember constantly being told to relax (I ask you – HOW?! I was almost semi-naked, surrounded by men and women I didn't know, I had a cold, I was about to be burned and, oh yes, a large, extremely heavy-looking porthole shaped device was poised above my face.)

"Has this machine ever broken?" I asked nervously.

"Not while in use," came the matter-of-fact reply. They added that they always do lots of checks.

I became aware of extremely narrow, red beams of light, obviously reflected from that long, narrow gap in the ceiling above me, and being reflected, or so it seemed through the circular device. (I hope no-one 'medical' is reading this with my poor medical terminology! They'd never believe I was a medical secretary a long time ago!)

All I could hear were people's voices throwing numbers at each other like 96.2, 318, etc. Absolutely meaningless to the layman (or woman). It sounded like I was lying in the middle of a bingo hall! Although I recognised similar numbers to those quoted appearing on the monitor screen. I couldn't look anywhere else!

Then they placed a 12 inch x 8 inch (approx – I don't know for sure, I wasn't able to measure it) thick, plastic sheet all across my chest, holding it in place with something like selotape and said they would take my 'image' first, for their records, which wouldn't be needed again for a week.

They explained that, in future, the whole process would be a lot quicker, as today's procedure was in order to tally everything with what the 'planning' had produced and there would be no need after this.

Without warning, they quietly disappeared into the other little room, telling me they would return momentarily. I believed them.

I lay there for a few seconds, all alone! Suddenly, the room lights came back on. I found it confusing that all should be illuminated now that they had finished sorting me out. I thought, at first, that it surely would have been better to have had the lights on to help them see things more clearly when they were working things out, but then I realised: the dimmed lighting made it more obvious where the beams were hitting me – at least I think that was the reason; as you know, I'm no doctor!

I heard quiet 'beeping' noises, coming from the machine. I was paralysed – not by the machine, by anxiety! They didn't have to tell me to keep still now. There was no way in the world I would move now – I didn't want to interfere with the functions in any way; I didn't dare cough even!

After about a minute, there was a sort of 'shooshing' sound from the machine, lasting a few seconds. Then it was over. The first part anyway. I was pleasantly surprised. The nurse had been right: I hadn't felt a thing. Oh joy! I thought that was it and expected to be sent home, but then the lights dimmed again and out they all came from their hidey place! One of them checked on me before leaving again saying, as he did, that there was only one more bit to go. The lights came on – I was left alone again. The big circular device moved away to make room for the other, rectangular-shaped unit, which slowly, quietly manoeuvred into place near my face. For about thirty seconds or so I heard the 'beeping' noise again, followed by 'shooshing' and then it really was all over.

The nurses appeared again. They lowered the bed in order to facilitate my sitting up and doing my poppers up, though I needed a little help with the shoulder ones.

As I was leaving, another nurse entered with an appointment card for me. She told me she had arranged for a meeting between myself and the doctor immediately after Thursday's session, to discuss the Tamoxifen drug. I thanked her and the others and returned to the cubicle to get dressed.

Whilst in the cubicle, I looked in the mirror and noticed what looked like a small black cross drawn in the middle of my chest – obviously where the original 'lost' tattoo was. On seeing it later, Simon called it a 'target'! Now I really was a target for his silly jokes!

I returned to the main waiting room and saw Ada reading the paper. I couldn't help but beam at her. She asked how it went and I responded by telling her that, in fact, I didn't know what I had been worried out – it turned out much better than I had expected – I really didn't feel anything; it was the thought of it, more than anything, that had been scary. At least I wouldn't be approaching the next session with a tentative demeanour!

2 pm: Debbie came round to our house, as arranged. We had tea and chatted for a while. She had had breast cancer, like myself. However, she now had secondary cancer in her leg and needed a walking stick. I noticed one of her arms was covered in a full-length 'tubigrip' which went all the way to her hands, with only the edge of her fingers showing. I asked how long she had to wear this for and she said 'forever'. I was stunned. Even more so when she explained the reason. Apparently, she had had her lymph glands removed (also like me), but because she overdid lifting heavy objects, six months after her operation she was informed she needed to wear this all the time. I told her I often find myself lifting fairly heavy objects, not because I'm disregarding medical advice, but because sometimes there just isn't anyone around to lift them for me – things like the linen basket when it's full of clothing, the washing basket when it's full of heavy, wet clothing, even food shopping, like milk and tins from the supermarket. She frowned and told me not to, not if I didn't want to end up the same way. I took her advice very seriously, at the time, but even now as I write this, I find I'm still in the same position of having to do these things myself. Simon's working away at the moment, in another county (temporarily) and Nick's at work. What do I do? I still have to buy food and do the washing. How can one nip next door to ask the neighbours to carry one's washing for them?

7.30: Attended my drama group's Casting Meeting. It was interesting to 'wear the shoe on the other foot' as they say. I usually audition, hoping to be cast. This time the actual decision was mine (though not mine alone)!

10/3/09:   9.15:   Zoe took me for my second treatment of radiotherapy, due at the same time of 9.50 am. She was smart enough to take some knitting with her to keep her occupied for the duration. Her latest project was a pair of multi-coloured socks, a sample of which she was wearing and proudly showed off!

I forewarned her to expect a possible delay, like yesterday, however that wasn't necessary as I was called in quite quickly this time. Plus I was much more relaxed about the whole thing, barring having to let out the odd cough again en route down the corridor, dressed in my usual little gown. I was greeted cheerfully by a different nurse. The tall radiographer was the only other nurse I recognised from yesterday. I sat on the bed as before, awaiting the oncoming thick steel 'porthole'. I commented to him, whilst he was busy locating my tattoo;

"If this thing falls on me, I've had it!", to which he replied

"There's not much chance of that – unless there's an earthquake!"

I couldn't be bothered to tell him that, in fact, England *has* experienced earthquakes, albeit comparatively minor ones. Instead I just coughed.

I noticed they were playing Abba music (from a cassette player – not the radiographers). It felt quite relaxing.

I wasn't as long in the treatment room as yesterday. He said it was because, this time, they viewed my image on the screen at the same time as the treatment. However, during the process, the 'clicky' noise I usually heard from the machine suddenly became more 'squeaky'. Also, at the end of the process, before I was told I could get up, I thought I could smell a tinge of burning, possibly coming from the machine (and hopefully not from me!). However, when I related this disconcerting news to the radiographer, he said he couldn't smell anything and smiled. Perhaps he was just used to it.

As I was retrieving my belongings from the chair, they told me that I didn't have a 'rest' day the following day, as originally scheduled. A rest day was just a day where I wouldn't need to attend a radiotherapy session. Instead, I could now attend the next session Wednesday of that week at 6.05 pm. I wasn't too happy but, as they commented, this would at least mean the entire process would be over a day earlier than planned. I agreed, and related the news to Zoe, who kindly offered to take me again.

On the way to her car (which, by the way, has a garden displayed on the parcel shelf...yes...that's what I said!), she remarked that she never saw one hunky doctor! I said that was because they were all in the treatment room – only it was just my luck that they saw me with just one boob!

Back home we had a coffee (one each). We discussed many things, as women do, one of which was the female menopause. (Have you noticed how all our troubles are caused by men? I.e: 'men'opause, 'men'struation, 'men'tal health...Anyway, to continue:) Apparently, one of her friends thought she was going through the menopause until, one year after chemo, her periods returned without warning! I was a bit perturbed to hear this, as I thought that that meant the same might happen to me....so I should probably be using contraception.... oh well....

That day it turned out that I must have passed my cold onto Nick (well, why should he be left out?!). It was so bad that it prevented him from cycling to work the next day.

Actually, I wasn't much better myself. I managed to drive to town to buy Gill a birthday present and post a large letter. However, in between the accumulating coughs and sneezes, my back suddenly began to hurt, which was unfortunate, as I had parked quite a way away from the main thoroughfare. I had only experienced this once or twice before in my life, so I was a bit of a stranger to this ailment, but it certainly helped me to sympathise with the many thousands of people who suffer from it regularly. Every step was agony. I began to feel very weak and tired – probably waiting for a long time in the post office queue didn't help much. I also felt very warm – especially inside the shops. By the time I eventually returned home I felt very lethargic, I didn't want to do a thing. I was just grateful I wouldn't be driving myself to the hospital that evening.

Zoe and I arrived at Oncology at 6.15. There was no-one at the reception desk, presumably because it was so late. Also, the tea kiosk and other shops were now closed, which was unfortunate, as we had planned on having a cuppa whilst waiting to be seen. But all was not lost. I told her that I knew a place where I thought we might be lucky in obtaining refreshment in another part of the hospital (trust me to know where to find food and drink!). So I led her down the corridor past the tea kiosk, turned left down another corridor, past another large, empty waiting area leading to a pair of double doors (which we thought, at first, were locked but, apparently, we just didn't use enough strength with the first push!), past many lifts (I told her it was quicker to use the stairs), up one flight of stairs (she was constantly concerned about whether I had enough energy for such a trek) and along another corridor until we finally reached a large restaurant area. We bought chocolate drinks in plastic cups with lids on and made our way back (via a lift this time) to the section with the double doors. Unfortunately, it turned out to be really locked this time! I said I knew where to go to try and get help, as we were opposite my old familiar 'chemo' territory. Again, the area was deserted, but we collared a passing nurse who said the only way back to Oncology was through the other double doors on the right which led to the outside area and the little covered walkway that led to Oncology. Dismayed, and with our drinks gradually getting cooler, we headed for those double doors. Just as we turned in their direction, we spotted a woman exiting the other double doors that we wanted! You should have seen us – a couple of women acting like teenagers running excitedly towards the doors, nearly spilling our drinks in the process, just to keep the woman from letting the doors close. We made it though! Don't know what that woman must have thought, but we were so relieved we didn't care. It actually brought back memories of school days but that's another book!

It wasn't long before I was seen. I got changed as usual and coughed all the way into the treatment room. After the first 'session', when the porthole moved away to be replaced by the other unit and the lights dimmed again, one of the nurses rearranged the 'mat' on my chest slightly. Then the second session began. I felt it slowly begin to slide off my chest. They obviously forgot to selotape it down this time. Eventually the inevitable happened – it slipped onto the floor whilst I was undergoing the treatment. I stayed motionless, controlling my desire to cough, my left arm still held in place in the air, head to one side, petrified! I didn't know what to do for the best, so I just did nothing. After the session had completed, the Indian radiographer came out, picked up the mat and told me that I had done the right thing in keeping completely still (probably to avoid them having to re-adjust my position more than anything else!). Then my coughing bout continued.

A few minutes later I returned to the empty waiting area to see Zoe still knitting her socks.

"I thought you might have knitted a whole outfit by now!" I exclaimed. Although I hadn't really been that long, I just felt like saying that!

I had offered her dinner as a 'thank you' for taking me but she declined as she had a few things to take care of that evening (apart from me!).

That evening I had a call from a fellow cancer sufferer, Nicky Coombes, who had also written a book about her experience called "I'm ill you know". Force Cancer Support had kindly passed on to her my details in order to get in touch with me to discuss the same. I was interested in several things, not least of all, I didn't want my efforts to be too similar to hers but I had discovered, on reading her book, that they weren't really, and told her so. I enquired as to her current health and we discussed where it was going. Then she told me about an incident that occurred after her book was finished, which she would have liked to have had included. So, Nicky – I hope you don't mind – I'll include it here for you (some of the facts may not be completely accurate, but you'll get the picture)!

During her unfortunate vomiting days (I can relate to them!), she awoke in the night feeling sick and urgently needed a container for the forthcoming contents. Her husband was in the bathroom so she fled, in the dark, to the kitchen, blindly feeling for a receptacle. Finally she found one, just in time, and vomited into the bowl. Afterwards, she could feel a warm, gooey mess oozing down her legs whilst she was still holding the bowl. She reached for the light, turned it on, and discovered she was holding a colander! Nicky, I wish you well.

12/3/09:   Don kindly took me to hospital today for my regular 9.50 appointment plus my brief meeting with a doctor, who turned out to be Dr Goodman's Registrar. We discussed my concerns over the Tamoxifen medication. She explained that the cancer they had discovered was the most aggressive – they number them in grades apparently: 1, 2 and 3, in order of severity, and apparently mine was the worst – number 3. So it was very strongly advised that I take the medicine for the next five years. I mentioned that I had read a customer's letter in the Amoena magazine (from where I bought my mastectomy bra) which detailed one of the side-effects she was starting to experience with the Tamoxifen – baldness! I told the young Registrar I was very concerned to read that, especially as I had only recently started to get my own hair back! She commented that the benefits of taking this drug would outweigh the risks. So I reluctantly agreed, adding that, as soon as I felt ill when taking it I would have to stop. I'd had a belly-full of pain the past year and just couldn't face going through it all again. As an after-thought, I asked if I would be able to take alcohol with it (I had missed my favourite "Baileys" drink!) and she confirmed that would be fine. So....not such a bad medicine after all!

So I bought the Tamoxifen with the prescription the Registrar had previously given me. It cost £7.10 but the pharmacist only had one bottle, saying I would be rung when they had delivery of the other three bottles for me. I went home and had one dose. Only then did I decide to read the accompanying leaflet. First was the obligatory information about not taking it if various conditions apply to you, i.e. if you are allergic to any of the ingredients, or if you are pregnant (no worries there), then an advisory notice concerning taking care when driving as it can cause changes in eyesight and light headedness, then came a list...a very long list, of possible side-effects. Apparently, very common (more than 1 in 10) subjects treated could suffer from hot flushes (I'm used to them now), vaginal discharge (not used to them), genital itching and abnormal vaginal bleeding; common side-effects (more than 1 in 100 subjects) could be: bone and tumour pain, fluid retention, increased risk of blood clots, deep vein thrombosis, pulmonary embolism (a blood clot in the lungs), light headedness, headache, changes in vision as a result of cataracts or changes to the cornea or retina, nausea (oh, not again), thinning of hair (ditto). Also possible (for which immediate medical attention must be sought – no kidding?): sudden shortness of breath, chest pain, coughing up blood, calf or thigh pain or swelling in the legs. Rare and very rare ones include cancer of the womb, liver cell damage, inflammation of lungs, difficulty breathing, and so on and so on......So....not much then..... And I was only worried about going bald again....

Foolishly or not, I just couldn't bring myself to have any more for now and decided to seek further medical opinions. Surely I could have a better quality of life now? And even if I didn't immediately get any of the side-effects, having to take it for <u>five years</u> surely increased the chances of getting them sooner or later within that period. I know it was supposed to help me but...at what cost!

I was now having to put the "Aqueous Cream BP" on the 'sunburnt' area of my chest morning and night. The previous night I got no sleep (nor did Simon, I suspect, from my continual coughing). I could feel the phlegm on my chest building up to an almighty crescendo of coughing every few minutes, inevitably keeping us both awake, so I resigned myself to sleeping on the guest bed in the spare room, which was actually quite comfortable, although I dare say my coughing could still be heard - the two rooms are separated only by a small landing area. I finally got to sleep around 6 a.m., when I heard our alarm go off in our bedroom. Simon got up and entered the guest room, informing me I could now go back into our bed. How kind!

Friday the thirteenth: I didn't catch on about the date until the day was over. Due to my cold and lack of sleep I just couldn't muster the strength for my fifth radiotherapy visit. I stayed in bed most of the day, coughing and sleeping when I could.

14/3/09:   Nick had another driving lesson.

7 pm: Simon went to his old employer, Marks and Spencer's leaving "do" at the inn over the road. He came home around 11.30 with a nice, little surprise for me – a big box of Belgian chocolates he had won as a raffle prize! He said he had a choice of those or a bottle wine but thought I would prefer the chocolates. He knows me well! (Made up for his insults anyway!)

15/3/09:   I was still suffering from the cold. I just couldn't shake off the cough. In spite of this, I managed to clear my throat and ring Gill to wish her a happy birthday. I feebly sang the 'Happy Birthday' song, at the end of which, she gayly announced "That's nice of you, but it isn't my birthday! It's on the 25th!"

"Oh," I replied, "Good job I didn't send you a card then!"

She laughed and said:

"Thanks anyway!"

"I'll give you your pressie tomorrow, when I see you – don't open it before your birthday, then!"

16/3/09:   Monday heralded the start of a bright, warm, sunny week, which cheered me up, despite the nagging phlegm on my chest. You would have thought that the radiation would have burnt through that and got rid of it!

Ada took me for my regular radiotherapy visit. We arrived ten minutes early and I barely had time to report my arrival to the receptionist, when a nurse came to collect me. Service or what! If only the other departments had been like that.   I didn't even have time to buy Ada a cup of tea as I had intended.

I went through the usual preparation by the radiographers as I was lying motionless on the bed. I kept perfectly still, as was required, moving not a muscle, for the few minutes it took to be 'radiated', at the end of which I commented to them that I could now play the part of a corpse on stage, as I have experience of remaining completely motionless!

As the weather was nice today, for a change, I asked if I would be able to sunbathe, but they naturally advised against such a pastime whilst I was undergoing such treatment. Regrettably, I saw the logic.

That evening Gill picked me up for another of my drama group's committee meetings at Jerry's house, which lasted the usual couple of hours.

17/3/09:   Zoe took me to hospital today (she apologised for calling late for me – something about losing her key, which turned out to be in the door of her car all along! Ah, Zoe! Queen of car gardens and lost property – not to mention colourful socks!).

She asked if I minded travelling to a nearby little town on the way back in order that she could buy some material and I said that was fine.

In radiotherapy, the nurses settled me into my position, as was the routine, and left the room, calling back to me:

"OK, we're going now!"

I replied

"Bye! Come back soon!"

They laughed and the older female nurse said they were going for a cup of tea!

"You'd better not!" I called to their backs as they disappeared into the little ante-room.

Soon after the machine had started to do its business, including the familiar 'beep beep' noises, it suddenly stopped. I knew it was too soon. The treatment was usually quick, but not that quick. I could hear one of the nurses in the other room instructing the other:

"Just press the button".

I held my breath.

The machine started again. Phew!

When they returned into my area, they explained that the machine sometimes gets 'too sensitive'. (Bit like me then.)

A little while later, Zoe and I arrived at the village for her quick bit of shopping, as arranged. She parked the car and I asked how far it was to the shop. She confirmed it was only a short walk away. I said I'd be fine with that. Once inside the quaint little haberdashery store, I browsed amongst the tableware items while Zoe spent some time choosing a lot of sewing and knitting material, occasionally seeking my opinion, which I was pleased to give, even if she didn't always agree! She was obviously a fairly regular customer, judging by the conversations she had with the shop assistants. The older shop assistant obviously had a bit of a cold, which Zoe remarked on. The woman related the story of its beginnings by attributing it to her husband who denied that he had passed it on to her. I felt like saying that I knew the feeling!

The other shop assistant measured up some more material for Zoe and it finally came to the time for her to pay for all the goods she had chosen. I stood near the doorway, waiting. Unfortunately, the poor woman, after frantically going through her large shopping bag, discovered that she had, in fact, left her credit card at home! She asked if they could keep the goods aside so she could pop back later that afternoon to pay for them and they agreed. I think she was a little embarrassed!

As we left the shop I nonchalantly remarked to the flustered shopper:

"It's just not your day, is it?!"

I tried to make her feel a little better by giving her a light lunch on the patio of our garden when we got back to our house (just tea and rolls). I managed to pull down the awning to keep me out of the sun (which was so frustrating because I usually hate sitting in the shade).

18/3/09:   Unemployment in the country had now passed the two million mark. So, Simon wasn't alone then.

8.40 am: Mary picked me up a little earlier than usual for my appointment, as she had another patient she had to take to hospital as well, for a different appointment. This meant I would arrive an hour early but never mind, I appreciated the lift.

The other female patient was a wheelchair user, so it was easier for her to sit at the front of the car (passenger side of course), while I sat at the rear. I was very aware of the folded wheelchair at the back of the 'People Carrier' vehicle bashing against the rear window throughout the long journey. It kept making me jump! The other patient remarked that it sounded like gunfire! I mentioned to Mary that it was going to give me a heart attack and added that it was therefore lucky that we were going to the right place! We all had a laugh anyway!

Mary dropped me off first, at Oncology, then took her other passenger to another department at the far end of the hospital. I read a newspaper while I waited.

Once I had been seen, I waited quietly in the fairly full waiting area. Every half hour or so, Mary returned to me, explaining that the other patient had had to attend another clinic, or have an X-Ray, and was I OK? I said I was and told her not to worry. She dashed back to her other patient.

Whilst I was waiting, I noticed one of the more mature (in age) receptionists walking awkwardly back to her desk, hanging tightly onto the hem of her long, grey skirt and laughing her head off. I asked what was wrong and she said something about catching the hem as she stood up from a seat, making it unravel. This was what had apparently brought about her hysterics! I smiled. Nice to know other people had bad luck too!

Then a tall, elderly gentleman appeared and sat two seats away from me. He reminded me a little of Santa Claus, with a demeanour and voice like the film actor James Robertson Justice. Shortly after arriving, he rose from his seat and asked if I wouldn't mind listening out for his name to be called, and letting staff know where he was, if that should happen. He was obviously going to the 'little boys' room'. I obliged, but his name was never called during my (long) time there!

Eventually Mary came back again to tell me it wouldn't be much longer now and that I should keep an eye out of the glass wall for her car, which would be near the entrance in a few minutes, ready to leave. Not long after, I spied it just where she said it would be, patient already on board, so I rushed out and took my lift home. Her patient was very apologetic for keeping me hanging around and even offered me a sweet! However, as it happened, I would be keeping Mary 'hanging around' the next day, when I would be seeing one of the Breast Care nurses for my prosthesis fitting. So my patience today would alleviate any guilt I might have tomorrow!

19/3/09: Half-way through my treatment! Hooray! I remember thinking how quickly one gets into a routine. I was actually getting used to rising early (for me!) in order to go to hospital every day to be burned!

I had my radiotherapy on time, as per usual, before going with Mary to see Sandra, the Breast Care nurse, on the second floor for my 10.30 appointment. Mary waited in the small Breast Care waiting room, which she said she was happy to do. She had a bit of time left before she had to bake some cakes for a WI function or some such thing that afternoon.

I had the fitting in the same little room where I had had my meeting with Annie a little while ago. She asked me how I was, especially after the mastectomy and I related a lot of the details of what had happened but that I was actually OK with my situation. I had brought my new mastectomy bra with me and tried it on with the prosthesis she had with her. The first one wasn't a good match for my other boob, so she obtained another one, which she inserted into the bra and it looked much better. She told me to put my loose-fitting jumper on to see how it looked then. It still looked good. She suggested I bring in more of my bras so that she can provide 'pockets' for them to ring the changes (mastectomy bras aren't cheap).

We discussed my concerns about the Tamoxifen medication and she said she would speak to Dr Goodman about it. She said if I was truly menopausal (not just temporarily chemo-induced for the moment), it might be possible to have a different medicine – something like Arimidex – which has less severe potential side-effects (hooray!).

She gave me advice about how to look after my new boob, for instance, it should be washed daily only in warm, soapy water (a bit like me then). It should last at least three years, generally, however if it is accidentally cut, I should cover it in clingfilm and the NHS would replace it free of charge (they normally cost £100 each). I was finally getting my moneysworth of paying my National Insurance for nearly forty years!

She put it in a nice blue, zipped container and placed that in a large box to take home with me.

2.30:   Nicki picked me up to attend Alan and Christine's Farm Auction which had started at 11.30. She couldn't get to me any earlier as she was at work in the local Doctor's Surgery until then. However, although we missed most of it, we managed to have a little look around at what was left (tractors, furniture, etc.) before being invited, by Christine, into the large farmhouse kitchen for some refreshments. I was surprised to see most of her family and friends already there and hoped it didn't look like Nicki and I had just come for the lovely spread of food! We left around four o'clock.

20/3/09:   9.50: Radiotherapy.

It was the day of the 'Carers Meeting' in a nearby village but Simon was unable to attend again, due to work commitments.

21/3/09:   Simon and I drove to a town in mid-Devon to see the shops and have a spot of lunch.

22/3/09:   'Mother's Day' today. I got a very apt card from Nick, basically outlying the trials of motherhood when you have a teenage offspring, who demands everything with little or no thanks. At least he obviously accepted that it was describing him, but did he doing anything about it? Did he change at all? Like hell!

Simon drove me to a pub just off the A35, where we had a drink each, although I just had a pineapple juice – the weather was too hot for alcohol! It was full of 'mums' having meals with their families. I wasn't bothered. I'd had a day out yesterday.

On the way back home, we popped into Tesco. Simon said he wanted to stay in the car. I picked a small trolley and studied the food in a section of the first aisle. I was particularly taken by the variety of Sushi and prawns on display but my concentration was being interferred with by the fact that my trolley seemed to keep moving towards me. I glanced at the wheels –were there brakes I didn't know about? Was something stuck in the wheels? Were they faulty? Was it a sloping floor? I carried on trying to decide what to buy but the trolley continued to push against me. I was flummoxed. How was that possible? It was as if it had a mind of its own and was trying to slowly run me over! I turned to my right and saw Simon pulling it from the side, grinning from ear to ear like a naughty schoolboy (I can see where Nick gets his attitude from!). I whacked him on his chest and shoulder with my hand and put some sushi into the trolley, telling him he could push it now!

Back home, I contemplated when I should start wearing my new boob. I thought it would probably be best to start wearing it after my radiotherapy had finished in a week's time, which was just as well, as I was (by now) getting fed up with having to hitch my 'cumfie' into place in order to keep it in line and even with my real boob! Not to mention the inconvenience of having to adjust oneself in public when the case arose!

I learned that day that Jade Goody had lost her cancer battle in the early hours of the morning, aged 27. A sobering thought: made worse by the fact that it happened on such a special day for mothers, which she was, having two young sons. At least my son was a fair age now, whatever happens.

23/3/09: Ada drove me to radiotherapy. Nothing much else happened today.

24/3/09: Hazel drove me to radiotherapy today.

At 2.30 Debbie visited again and stayed for a little while.

25/3/09: Today was Gill's birthday (not the 15th, as I had previously thought!) She rang later to tell me she had been good (a challenge for such a worldly woman – sorry Gill!). She had waited until today to open my little present for her – a candle inside a circular glass container inside which were little flowers; it probably has a correct name but you know me and terminology!

I had an afternoon appointment for my radiotherapy today (2.40). I was driven by a young, dark-haired woman called Rowena of Hospiscare (that is Rowena who worked for Hospiscare – what I just wrote sounded like a medieval title!) just before two o'clock. Unfortunately, the immediate car park was completely full, with cars queuing for spaces. Rowena's was one of them. She dropped me off by the walkway so that I wouldn't be late and said she would try and find a space.

Talk about a small world: I was walking back from the tea kiosk carrying a small (and I mean small) packet of Minstrel chocolates, when I noticed Debbie queueing at reception, with her family (her husband and one of her daughters). They sat next to me and we chatted until I was called. Rowena was obviously still looking for a parking space.

I got changed as usual and, when I took a seat in the additional waiting area, I saw Debbie and her family had taken up most of the seats!

"Are you following me?!" I asked and sat on one of the last chairs, with a good view of the main waiting area.

Inside the treatment room, shortly afterwards, the radiographers asked if I was OK or whether I had been experiencing any pain. I said no. However, I had noticed that I was getting a little spotty around the designated area and wondered if it was due to the abundance of cream I had been plastering onto it twice daily. They said no, it was a perfectly normal reaction to radiotherapy treatment, which relieved me (the news, not the radiotherapy).

I noticed they had finally changed the CD during treatment. Instead of listening to Abba, I was being burned to the tune of "I can make you feel good"! Really?

When it was time to go, I couldn't see Rowena in the waiting room so I went outside into the car park. I ambled through the first few rows of cars before I spotted her car and saw her reading at the wheel! Apparently, she just missed out on one space, to which another driver had beaten her, so she gave up and decided to stay where she was – parallel to the row, blocking some cars! I didn't blame her.

I invited her back to my house after, as I did all my chauffeurs. She accepted.

She made an interesting remark whilst there. On seeing one of the (many) photos I had on display of Nick, she commented on how she thought he looked like David Cassidy! Now, as it happens Heather and I used to have a huge crush on that seventies pop idol and, of course, I couldn't really see the similarity. Still, if that meant Nick looked like a handsome pop star, I won't argue with that.

Whilst we chatted, I discovered that her husband owned one of the local food companies in league with some famous lord or other. So you see, you never know who you're talking to!

26/3/09:   I was very tired today. I think the radiotherapy must have finally started to kick in.

I was driven to hospital by another Hospiscare drive, Jim. He was a large man of mature years, with a white beard. Luckily there were plenty of car parking spaces today – probably because it was morning, rather than afternoon. "Don't tell Rowena!" I said, relating her lack of success in parking the previous day.

I was called for my treatment, leaving him to read the national newspaper in the main waiting area.

In the treatment room, they took another image of me, which added just a few seconds to the overall time!

Nothing much else happened that day that didn't happen before.

27/3/09:   It was the day of Nick's long-awaited driving test. I noticed he had been trying to hide his anxiety about it in recent days (I overheard his phone calls to his friends). However, he needn't have worried – around 9 am the DSA rang to apologise that the test would have to be postponed due to the lack of an examiner. Nick was relieved yet frustrated at the same time. I had to re-arrange it for the following week and hope that his driving instructor could make that day. He could, but he asked me to obtain a claim form from the DSA for the loss of pay for both him and Nick, who had booked half a day off work with no pay. I had to organise all this on my return from hospital. Ada took me today.

In the treatment room I made myself comfortable on the bed as usual and they started to swing it into position, followed by manoeuvring the large equipment round into place.

It prompted me to comment:

"It feels good when you swing the bed round into position but feels bad as you bring this steel porthole-shaped thing into place!"

"Is it because it's on top of your face?" they asked. Well, they knew the answer to that!

I was very weak and tired today. I yawned to and from the hospital in Ada's car. I think she was worried about it being catching – especially while she was driving! I couldn't help it.

She got me home then I slept most of the day. I don't know where it came from, I just had to do it!

Karen, the Avon lady, called this evening. I had to tell her I couldn't afford anything this time. Of course, the splendid makeup provided by Force's 'Look Good, Feel Good' session had meant I was in no desperate need for makeup for a long time anyway, so I told her! Fortunately, she understood.

28/3/09: Simon decided to start a 'sock fight' with me this morning as he was getting dressed. He does that sometimes (sock fighting. He always gets dressed.).

We were due to see Alan in his local village's pantomime production of 'Strictly Coombe Dancing' and that's not a spelling mistake! To prepare for attending the afternoon matinee I washed my hair but, unfortunately, at this moment in time, it was still spiking up after a wash, making me look very cool if I was a young lad! Nothing I did worked to flatten it so I just had to accept it – I hadn't worn my wig for ages and didn't want to revert to that again. So I donned some dangly earrings and a bit of makeup. However, I was wearing trousers, so the whole ensemble did little to stop me from looking like a lesbian! No offence to lesbians, however one doesn't really want to be mistaken for one if one isn't, if you know what I mean! So I made sure I was always near Simon, holding his hand, that kind of thing!

29/3/09: British Summer Time began. I'd put the clocks forward the night before.

30/3/09: My last day of radiotherapy treatment – hooray!

Ada took me again for my 9.50 appointment. On arrival, I handed her a small cheque donation for Hospiscare, only sorry I couldn't afford more.

The advice board behind the reception desk stated there would be a fifty minute delay. Oh dear. So I bought a cup of tea for each of us and was just starting to read a magazine when my name was called. It was only two minutes after my usual time (9.52) but evidently they had managed to sort out the machine that had been creating problems. I was apparently quite lucky, the radiographer informed me, because they had only recently sent a couple of patients home.

I had my treatment, bade them all farewell (a more cheerier one than usual!) and returned to Ada in the waiting area. My tea was cold!

CHAPTER THIRTY-FOUR

Thanks for the Mammories! (Life Goes On....)

So...I'd been diagnosed with breast cancer, had a breast partially removed, had chemotherapy for six months, had a breast completely removed, had radiotherapy for three solid weeks (bar weekends) and now....well now I had to await the outcome of my blood test to determine my 'menopausal' state, which would have a bearing on which medicine I would need to continue to take for the next five years!

As it turns out, I <u>am</u> menopausal. I sounded so overjoyed at the news on the telephone, that the GP's receptionist told me it was nothing to sound particularly happy about. But I disputed that, telling her:

"Yes it is. That means I can have the medicine with less severe side-effects, I'll have no more period pains, and it also means I haven't been having these hot flushes for nothing!" I think she understood.

Life is, sort of, getting back to normal for now. Though I suffer a little pain at bedtime from the tissue inside the boobless part of my chest which, I have on good authority, is more than likely due to inflammation from the radiotherapy on the scar tissue and which should go sometime. Michelle, another Hospiscare nurse, asked if I take paracetamol. I replied "No. I just turn over!"

Debbie also advises me that I shall probably remain 'sunburnt' on my boobless area for years to come! Thanks Debbie!

I am not allowed to wear deodorant, either, for at least four weeks, so thank heavens we don't have many hot days in this country! I still have to use non-perfumed soap. I also understand I'll probably suffer from fatigue for a while and my GP said that, as my body has been "through the mill" this past year, I probably won't be completely back to normal for at least a year. Will anyone notice the difference?!

Socially, things are still active, even if I'm not! We had our first rehearsal of our forthcoming Agatha Christie play on 2nd April (now I've finished this book I can concentrate on producing the programme for it) and I've signed up for the Cancer Research 'Race for Life' due to take place on 5th July (I'm going with Zoe – if I have the energy). I mentioned this to Irene, making a passing comment about taking the opportunity to use the occasion to not only raise money for cancer research but also to, perhaps, publicise this book in the process. She suggested I wear some sort of banner or poster around me with a slogan like newspaper headlines have, only in my case it would be 'Lost Tit – read all about it!' (her words, not mine!). Thanks Irene!

I'm contemplating when and how I can return to work, but a lot depends on the outcome of a meeting I'm having with the surgeon, Mr Ferguson, in August regarding possible reconstructive surgery. From what I understand, one doesn't initially have nipples at the first stage of the process. However, whilst waiting to pick Nick up from work recently, I noticed a tall, elegant white statue of a 'Venus'-like woman, carrying a bow or something (was she Amazon, I wondered?) Her toga-style dress draped down her shoulders to reveal one of her breasts, which had no nipple. Well they don't, do they? Statues. So I'd be able to say I had something in common with elegant statues! Though that's where the similarity ends!

Before that meeting I've got a follow-up meeting in May with Dr Goodman, presumably to check on my condition following the radiotherapy. Whilst there, I'll be having a meeting with Research Nurses of the Clinical Trials Unit to discuss my possible participation in their Diet and Lifestyle Study for the next five years (which involves form filling – I'm used to that now, blood tests and urine samples) to, hopefully, help others. I've also been invited to become a member of the NHS Trust and am seriously considering it, time permitting. But I do have a play to finish. I stopped work on my last play "No Such Agency" in order to write this book. So I think I'll get back to that now....before I end up writing the sequel to this book, should I go ahead with the next lot of treatment! Happy days!

And to anyone who has, in any way, experienced breast cancer, or thinks they might have it, of course you don't have to take my advice, but – for what it's worth – First: Don't listen to anyone other than your doctor if you suspect a lump (husbands can be just as scared as you) and Second: there *IS* life after cancer (or at least, after the diagnosis), and during. And ultimately, even if you're not lucky enough to be surrounded by many caring family members, friends, organisations, all you need is a little faith. I'm sure mine helped me......God be with you.

AN UPLIFTING EXPERIENCE
By
Jan Guscott

People deal with bad news in different ways. You can either let it get you down or look at the positive aspects. I chose the latter. After all, when there's not much you can do about it, why mope? Instead, I decided to write about the experience, in the hope that, above all, no-one would leave the diagnosis as late as I did and, therefore, avoid the intense treatment! However, such treatment in itself can have its funny side, believe it or not. Humour creeps in in strange places. Or perhaps I just always find the funny side of things!

I wrote this book in much the same way that I usually write my books and plays – not knowing how it will end (and I still don't)! I hope you never have to go through what I did but, even if you do, I hope you enjoy it (this book, not the cancer treatment). Anyway, I always say a little bit of good comes out of everything, if you look hard enough – for instance, I'm donating a percentage of this sale to *Cancer Research UK!* So thank you for your purchase and happy reading!

About the Author

Jan Guscott has always loved writing and acting. On moving to Devon, she joined a local Writers' Circle. She convinced the group to read a sample of her then latest play (a comedy called "Chain Reaction"), and was so impressed with their interpretation that, seeing there were no local amateur dramatic facilities in the area, she decided to start her own drama group, even though she had dismissed the idea when it was first put to her by her previous drama group in Ascot (CADS).

Together with Don, a fellow Writers' Circle member, and after doing a fair bit of research on her new home town, she penned the drama group's opening performance "Stall Trek - Pennies From Devon". The local Mayor introduced the group and they performed the play to a full house.

Jan's previous work includes one of her first books "Destiny", a pantomime called "Pantocourt" and a play called "The Uninvited", which was showcased at the Progress Theatre. BBC Radio 2 was interested in a romantic, wartime play of hers ("A Time to Remember") as was a London film company, for whom she wrote a romantic thriller screenplay called "Nine Days".

When suddenly stricken by Breast Cancer in 2008, Jan decided to put aside work on her current play ("No Such Agency") in order to share her experience with others in the hope that her suffering wouldn't be entirely in vain, at the same time donating a percentage of sales to Cancer Research UK.

Jan is a qualified Mental Health Act Administrator and, hitherto, has worked as a Legal and Medical Shorthand P.A. Secretary since the age of 16. Jan likes to travel (Europe, USA, Canada) and is entering the "Race for Life" for Cancer Research also participating in Clinical Trials for the next five years.

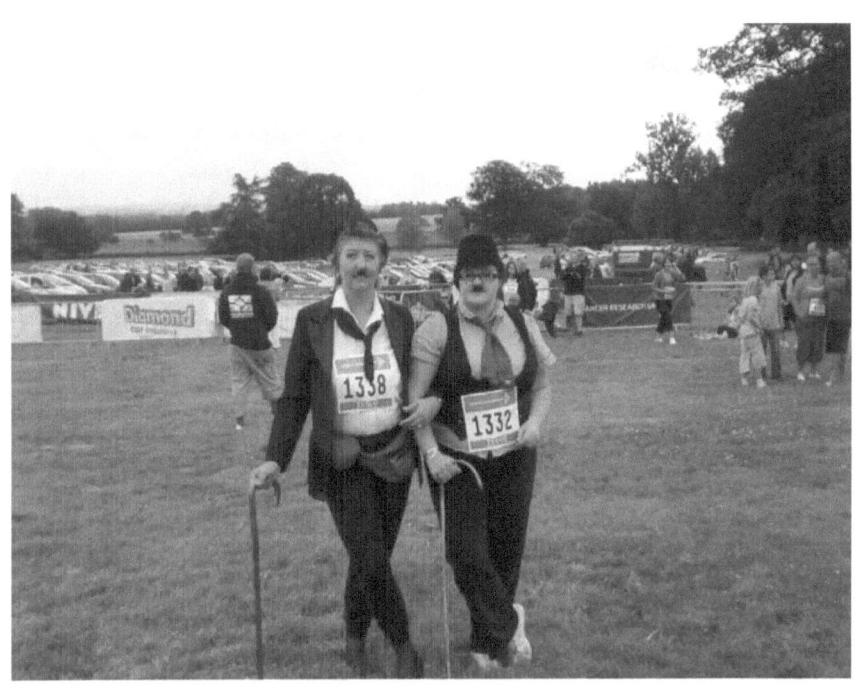

5th July 2009

Myself and friend Zoe as a "couple of Charlies" at the onset of the
Race For Life for Cancer Research UK, Killerton Gardens, Devon.

[Photo by S.R. Guscott]